"This is an empowering book that makes the endless details manageable - from her 41years of experience. I felt like I was learning from an old friend over a cup of tea. This should be required reading for doctors, health professionals, MS patients and their families."

–Sharon Baldacci, MSer, Author of *A Sundog Moment*

"This book contains some of the best info about MS and how to deal with it that I have found anywhere. It was so interesting that I read it straight through in one sitting. I have MS and I think everyone with it should read this book! I appreciated her honestly and humor."

–Amazon, Verified Purchase

"I'm recently diagnosed and needed a book that offered the inside scoop from someone who's been there. This book is very accessible and written in a style that feels like chatting with a close friend. I learned a lot and feel like I have a better handle on what I could be facing."

—Amazon, Verified Purchase

""Debbie Petrina has managed to improve her no-nonsense, been-there-done-that guide to navigating the often choppy waters of multiple sclerosis. For personal advice without the unnecessary puffery, it's just what the doc ordered."

—Dave Bexfield, founder of www.ActiveMSers.org

"Managing MS provides practical and meaningful guidance for people living with MS as well as for their family and friends. In addition, caregivers and health care providers can learn ways to understand someone who has been diagnosed with MS."

–Ellen Friedman, Physical Therapist, Scottsdale AZ

"Good common-sense advice; not preachy. Very user-friendly."

–Jeffrey Fisher M.D., (retired, Consultants in Internal Medicine, Glendale, AZ)

"This book is INCREDIBLE and easy to read. The clinical information and personal experience provided not only answers key questions but reassures readers that they are not alone."

–Sandy Dow, Neuro-Trauma ICU RN, Pittsburgh, PA

"I learned so much about MS and also about the human spirit that allows us to cope with whatever we are presented with. Debbie writes in a style that is not only easy to read, but also educates & offers inspiring ways to think about and face life's challenges successfully & gracefully! She doesn't hype management strategies, nor does she make claims about unproven treatments or therapies."

–Barb Lambing - Registered Dietitian, retired

"Debbie Petrina's book, Managing MS, is the perfect "bible" for those of us who deal with this condition and our families, whether newly diagnosed or battling for many years. As a leader in MS and fitness I highly recommend this book as part of a MS management protocol along with a solid fitness program."

–David Lyons B.S., C.P.T., Founder MS Fitness Challenge/Optimal

MANAGING MS

MANAGING MS

A Roadmap to Navigate Multiple Sclerosis

Second Edition

Debbie Petrina

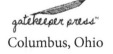
gatekeeper press™
Columbus, Ohio

Managing MS: A Roadmap to Navigate Multiple Sclerosis

Published by Gatekeeper Press
2167 Stringtown Rd, Suite 109
Columbus, OH 43123-2989
www.GatekeeperPress.com

Library of Congress Control Number: 2021946158

ISBN (paperback): 9781662917943
eISBN: 9781662917950

This book is dedicated to my MS peers and friends.

Contents

Foreword

Debbie Petrina's guidebook on Multiple Sclerosis is an inspirational, first-hand encounter of living with MS. Patients and physicians would benefit from this actual account of Debbie's story. As a Nurse Practitioner, the book opened my eyes to the effects of the disease on my patient's lives and their medical needs. This is not a textbook read.

If you are a patient of MS, you would benefit from reading this book. You may laugh, cry, and come to terms with the current life of MS through Debbie's eyes. I would highly recommend reading this wonderful, exceptional book to help guide any professional or patient through the incredible journey of the life of a person with MS.

Debbie's strength and courage with this disease should be an inspiration to continue the fight to survive MS.

Diane L. Perry, NPC
Consultants in Internal Medicine
Glendale Arizona

Preface

Enjoy the ride today, but keep aware of what's best for your journey.

Overall health and wellness became a primary approach for handling multiple sclerosis in recent years—it now includes *both* medical and non-medical ways. Before then, the emphasis was primarily on the medical ways to treat MS. Medical treatments are still too often thought to be the primary way to handle multiple sclerosis, but thankfully, this is changing.

I wrote the first edition of this book in 2011 and listed "My Ten Commandments" a.k.a. health and wellness, as my primary way of managing MS. It is gratifying that multiple sclerosis is being approached in the same way. All the parts of a car must always be attended to continuously, if the car is going to operate and reach its destination.

At the present time, here's the destination for MS: Until a cure is discovered, or restorative abilities to damaged areas are found, it is paramount that a person with MS live with their primary focus to be preventing as much damage to the nervous system as possible.

There are many aspects of health and wellness that include, but are not limited to:

- Physical Wellness—such as sleeping, eating, and exercising properly; watching your weight; avoiding the use of tobacco, drugs, and excessive alcohol consumption.

- Social Wellness—having healthy, positive interpersonal relationships with family, friends, pets and others.

- Spiritual Wellness—finding meaning and purpose in life. This may or may not include religion.

- <u>Emotional Wellness</u>—understanding our feelings and emotions and knowing action plans to follow when needed.

- <u>Intellectual Wellness</u>—maintaining cognitive stimulation to prevent mental stagnation. It is a lifelong process of mental challenges and creativity.

Medical treatments are an integral part for sure, but they can't get us to our destination alone. They also need to be attended to frequently.

One must think of managing MS in both the short and long term. After all, there is no cure yet and nobody knows when this will happen. We have one body; we need to protect it, be proactive, and make prudent choices. For example, every drug that is taken has to be processed through the liver. What are the risks vs. benefits of any drug we take regularly after 10, 20, 30 or 40 years? Diet and exercise help define our health. It's rational to nurture it.

Is it easy? Quite frankly, no. It takes a tremendous amount of grit, discipline, determination, and control. Now in my seventh decade of life, I am slowing down; yet I'm still managing MS in the same manner, quite well and independently.

I know two things. First, if I didn't practice good health and wellness, my MS would be so much worse. Second, if/when that breakthrough for remyelination or a cure arrives, I'm in great shape for it. How did I do it?

This book is a roadmap of an MS journey, a roadmap for all to navigate MS. Why should someone read this book?

- Less-complicated explanations reduce confusion; a person will lose their way. I strive to honestly help others with MS find their way.

- Too much information from countless sources cause frustration. Focus and direction are lost, or the wrong pedals are pushed. I want to offer credible guidance and reassurance.

- Multiple sclerosis through the vantage point of a patient is different as compared to the view from a medical professional or non-MSer. Health care professionals, patients and others need to understand each other.

While it is estimated that one million persons in the U.S. alone have MS (Source: National MS Society), millions of others without it also have to live with it or work with it. It is my hope that everyone interacting in the MS arena (i.e., patients, family/friends, and health professionals/workers) will obtain guidance and knowledge as well. It helps make life for an MSer easier.

Sincerely,

Debbie Petrina

Acknowledgments

Barry Hendin, M.D., thank you for your review and thoughts of my book, as well as the support you gave me being my neurologist for the past 16 years. Jeffrey Fisher, M.D., many thanks for your complete review, suggestions and corrections to the *Managing MS* draft and being my incredible internist for twelve years. Sitting with me at my kitchen table while discussing the book meant the world to me. Angela Felix, D.O., my PCP for the past eight years, I am grateful not only for your help and support, but for your desire to honestly learn about MS in addition to me personally to understand best how to offer treatment. Ellen Friedman, my physical therapist for four years, thank you for your friendship, the help you have personally given me for managing my MS, and the thorough review/recommendations of the initial draft of my book.

Rita Wilson, dear and supportive friend since before my MS began, an accomplished English professor and author—thank you for your extensive editing, review and constructive critique of my manuscript. Your immediate response to calls and texts will always be cherished. Equally cherished are the contact, support and friendship throughout the decades from Pauline Morgan, Debbie Chipman and Beverly Flaherty (and kids!) since our early school days together. And my dear aunts Dorothy Lakly, Donna Lakly—your support, wit, and humor throughout my life is priceless. Special acknowledgements wouldn't be complete without including neighborhood friends, a huge part of my survival arena. Thank you, Lynn Franklin, my childhood friend and an accomplished author, for introducing me to the world of publishing.

Sincere appreciation to those that read my initial manuscript and gave me their honest feedback: Diane Perry, NPC (Nurse Practitioner at Consultants in Internal Medicine); Sandy Dow, (Neuro-Trauma ICU RN);

Anne Mageras (President, Pennsylvania Keystone Chapter, NMSS) Ellen Langas (President and Founder, Nousoma Communications, Inc.); Barbara Lambing (retired Registered Dietitian, friend); MS buddies Renée Newman, Gerry Markle, Jacqueline Dawso; and the main players of my survival team—Mum and stepdad, Helen and Lee Schlabach, only a phone call away; brother John Furjanic who put his life on hold when support was badly needed; sister, Suzi Furjanic, husband, Den and son, Chad for always being there for everything.

Finally, I am grateful to all of the people with MS, my MS peers and friends, The National MS Society, and others I have spoken to about MS, as you have helped me as much as I helped you. This book could not have been written without you.

PART I

WHO IS DEBBIE, THE AUTHOR?

A Mouth and a Brain

(May 18, 2011)

In 1980, 41 years ago, I walked into a neurologist's office with weird things happening to me. Four years later, my diagnosis was confirmed.

I have a mouth and a brain. I have always said that I use them both to get what I need or want. Through the years as I became more disabled, I have used my mouth and my brain to figure out ways to manage my life and stay as independent as possible.

Today I went to Best Buy to get a wireless mouse for my notebook. I called the store first to make sure they had what I wanted and asked them to hold one for me at customer service. When I got there, I called them and explained that I had driven with hand controls since I don't walk and didn't have my wheelchair with me. Could someone bring it out to the car for me? —I had the exact amount in cash for payment.

The clerk explained it was store policy that employees were not allowed to leave the store. This was the first time that this had ever happened to me; when I had done this at other places I was always accommodated. Hmm—plan B. Okay, not to worry, I said. I will grab a Good Samaritan to get it for me. It was only $16 so I didn't have much to lose.

There are good people in the world. After eyeing a few passersby, I motioned to an older couple and explained my situation. They were happy to help. I graciously thanked them.

Mission accomplished.

In the Beginning

It wasn't always this easy, and I didn't always have this attitude. In 1980 I was 25, full of life, hopes and fun. Then the bomb fell.

I walked out of a sales presentation and noticed that when I got into my car my left shoe was missing. It was lying in the parking lot twenty feet away. Other strange things were happening to me prior to this incident, but this was the ultimate. I drove straight to the hospital in a little town in Pennsylvania called Altoona, and was told to go to a neurologist in Pittsburgh ASAP. I shook and cried during the whole two-hour trip.

Forty-one years ago, there were no CAT scans, MRIs, or visual evoked response (VER) testing. VER testing is a diagnostic tool that measures if nerve impulses are normal. I was asked a series of questions, checked clinically in the office by walking and doing some other things, and then admitted into the hospital for a myelogram. A myelogram is a test to look for problems in the spine, by taking X-rays of the spine after dye is injected into the spinal canal through a thin needle. I was told I had an infection in my spinal column and sent home.

I suffered two weeks of excruciating headaches from not being told to lie down for 24 hours after the myelogram. The neurologist (Dr. Pathetic) put me on a high dosage of prednisone, never bothering to mention that I could have insomnia as a side effect as well as many other side effects. He said I had an infection in my spinal cord and that it would slowly go away. There was nothing else to do. I slept an average of two hours a night, went back to work, and nearly became an alcoholic.

At that time, few people knew anything about MS. I brought it up to my family after reading an old encyclopedia, but everyone denied it. It was my nerves, they said. I was overworked and was too young to have anything wrong with me. There was no internet, little awareness, and scant literature on the subject. The only reason I knew about MS was because the next-door neighbor where I grew up had it.

I felt alone and terrified. My usual discipline, self-control, and logic were lost; anxiety and stress took over. I had trouble balancing, my left leg was weak and heavy, my left toes were cold; I couldn't warm them up after running hot water over them. I began writing these and other bizarre happenings down in a journal. The strange symptoms lasted ten months and then all mysteriously went away except for an itching sensation in my left forearm.

But MS stuck in the back of my mind because of something I had read in that old encyclopedia. I had the Babinski sign. The Babinski sign is a test the neurologist will perform in the office. The bottom of the foot is scraped and, in normal people, the big toe will involuntarily turn down. If it turns up, it is an indication that there is a neurological disorder. My toes had turned up. I also had the Lhermitte's sign— another sign of a neurological dysfunction. This is when you lower you head so that your chin touches the chest, a tingling shock-like sensation zips down the back or body. The neurologist never responded to me when I asked about them. Again, he just said I had an infection in my spinal cord, and not to worry about it. I was too naïve and scared to press further.

Two months after I delivered my son in 1983, it all started again, but differently. I began wetting the bed. My balance and leg coordination were affected. I lost almost all the sight in my left eye. Deep down inside I knew I had MS but my life at the time was too complicated to go for a diagnosis. My husband had lost his job, and by year-end I had lost mine too. Both his parents had passed away. Then I started a new job. My son was now an active one-year old. During that one year, the intense stress from all these major life events was breaking down all my main body functions. It was time to do something.

So, in 1984, four years after the initial onset of symptoms, I called a cousin who was a nurse and asked about a recommendation for a new neurologist. He diagnosed me immediately. I had the *multiple* symptoms

4

in *multiple* parts of the nervous system. Now, the *multiple* occurrences, the presence of optic neuritis, and positive findings of a new visual evoked response test made his conclusion that I had MS. I was actually relieved! I finally had answer to my suspicions confirmed. I could go forward and figure out how to deal with this.

Unfortunately, at that time there still was very little awareness of MS. It was a gloom-and-doom picture of a person who eventually ended up twisted in a wheelchair. It's that "Jerry Lewis thing, isn't it?" everyone asked. Family told me to get a second opinion.

Instead, I went to the local chapter of the National Multiple Sclerosis Society (NMSS) office. It was very small, but welcoming. They gave me some basic brochures about MS, the names of a couple of books that I later ordered through a bookstore, and a name and number of another young woman that had it (after getting her permission to be contacted.) Her name was Cathy.

**

Cathy was my saving grace. We were about the same age and both of us had a young child the same age. We clicked instantly, sharing stories and feelings. When I told her about my cold toes, she told me how she always had to wear a sock on her left foot. We were phone buddies for years. Relief was spelled "P-e-e-r".

Beyond my chats with Cathy, there was nobody to teach me the ropes. I was on my own. I read, I experimented, and then I got involved with the local chapter of the National MS Society and met more people with MS. I used my mouth, my brain, and as my great aunt used to say "used my intelligence."

Today in 2021, it's incredible how much information, awareness, assistance, research, medication, support and access available to folks diagnosed with MS. Learning the ropes is easier for persons with MS today, but it still is an overwhelming process one has to experience, be taught and learned. It's not the gloom-and-doom picture it used to be, but it's not the perky bowl of cherries that's often pictured either. It will take time and patience.

I am considered an advanced MSer[1] and the so-called worst-case: the one in four or five who ended up in a wheelchair. However, the progress in all aspects of MS has been so tremendous in the past forty years, I'm sure those getting diagnosed today will statistically have a better prognosis.

**

I was only 25. I am now 66, married 43 years, have a 38-year-old son, and many stories to tell of my struggles and successes. I still drive, lead a productive life, and weigh less than 115 pounds. People who look at me in my scooter tell me how good I look and ask what type of accident I had.

That's what this book is about—learning the ropes from someone who has MS. The countless things I learned over decades and then how I managed. How I managed myself, my MS, my life. This book is opinions, trials and errors, experiences, and judgments. So much was learned from extensive interaction with others throughout the years.[2] I am still learning and will continue to do so.

There are no absolute rights or wrongs. What works for one, may or may not work for another—something that I will repeat many times throughout this book.[3]

Truthfully, I hate MS—it's interfering, unpredictable, and invisible in so many ways. I didn't have a choice about getting it, but I did have a choice about whether I was going to let it control me or manage my life.

You can, too! But first, there are a few things you should know about me—outlined in the next chapter— as you read this book.

---

[1] For many years, we used to refer to persons with MS as "MSers".

[2] Medical information, symptoms, drugs, etc. throughout this book have been properly researched from sources listed in *Resources/Bibliography*. Every effort has been made to provide accurate and dependable information.

[3] I do not personally endorse products or companies mentioned in this book.

Information about My Background

Okay, so I started off by telling my story. But before continuing, I want to tell you something about my background. The point is that what I learned and how I manage(d) are not only my personal experience of living with MS for 41 years; they also are a result of interactions with thousands of peers and persons associated with MS.

<u>I have been a</u>:

- Trained peer counselor by the National Multiple Sclerosis Society (NMSS). I counseled hundreds of persons dealing with MS for 15 years for the Society, and have continued to counsel other peers confidentially to the present through referrals from acquaintances and personal health-care personnel.

- Monthly group leader for the NMSS for 11 years.

- Volunteer for MS Events, like the NMSS MS Walk.

- Member of the chapter services committee for the (then) Allegheny District Chapter in Western Pennsylvania.

- Frequent speaker to newly-diagnosed groups; caregivers/family groups; medical staff on behalf of the NMSS; hospital staff.

- MS blogger. Constant researcher/participant of MS news, publications, social media, etc.

- Participant in workshops by pharmaceutical companies (EMD Serono, Pfizer, Genzyme).

I also earned my Bachelor of Science in Business Administration degree in 1976 from Duquesne University in Pittsburgh, Pennsylvania. My major was marketing and minor was statistics. I worked for two major banks for over ten years in finance, research, sales and management. These skills have been invaluable throughout the years as I researched, analyzed, and engaged myself with MS.

Now let's take a look at My Ten Commandments I follow in my life...

My Ten Commandments

———————

There is no magic pill or shot you can take to make it all go away. It takes work, discipline, dedication, attitude, and common sense to take care of yourself. This is a lifetime illness. Until there is a cure for multiple sclerosis the goal is to stay healthy, prevent new attacks, and prevent disability.

How do I do it?

1. Rest/sleep.

I make the time to rest at various intervals throughout the day, especially since I wake up once or twice at night to pee and don't always fall back to sleep right away. I take an afternoon nap to lie flat, and resort to the recliner to elevate my feet to help the edema (swelling). I make sure I sleep; I *make* myself sleep. I have used sleeping pills for over 35 years when needed. Good sleep and rests are a must. They rejuvenate and heal the body, reduce anxiety, fatigue, and depression and keep one's resistance up.

- Check out:

    "The Complete Guide to Insomnia - How You Can Manage It"
    https://howtosleep.co.uk/guides/the-complete-guide-to-insomnia

    "The Power of Sleep"
    https://time.com/3326565/the-power-of-sleep

- Sleeping prescriptions are discouraged. However, they are often necessary as an interim, permanent, or last resort with MS/other chronic conditions.

2. Eat properly.

I follow no special diet, eat what's good for me and avoid what's not. Truthfully, I don't eat a lot. Balance, variety, and quantity are key. Lots of fresh fruits and veggies (low in calories, good fiber). A mix of fish, poultry, pork, beef, pasta every week (balance of protein, omega-3's, carbs…). Small meals several times a day (keeps the stomach feeling full). Very limited sauces, gravies, butter (less calories); the plainer, the better (lots of seasoning gives me gas and/or causes me to retain water). Cook, broil and grill at home—I eat out only occasionally. I always drink water, except for a mug of coffee in the morning or green tea later in the day. No dairy products (they cause bloating and nausea for me, and are binding). Instead, I take calcium, and acidophilus for 'good' bacteria. I don't deprive myself of potato chips or goodies—I just put a strict limit on them. No fast food unless I'm desperate. Liquor? I've had a cocktail or wine many evenings for years and will not give that up! I enjoy it. My doctor tells me to go for it, as long as it's in moderation.

3. Keep the weight down.

Obviously, we all know it's healthier, but equally important: *it puts less strain on the body which is challenged by fatigue 24/7 and makes it easier to exercise.* By keeping my body weight under 115 pounds, others can pick me up when necessary and I can maneuver myself easier. When I quit smoking 35 years ago, I gained 15 pounds. I bought a book that was popular at that time called *The Rotation Diet* that taught me how to eat right and how to increase my metabolism while I lost weight. I lost those 15 pounds in three weeks, and never put it back on. I learned that a slab of butter is 100 calories, as is a slice of American cheese or only one tablespoon of salad dressing. It was hard, and it took a lot of discipline, but it was worth it.

4. Exercise all day, every day.

This is one of the most important things a person with MS can do. I have been a swimmer all of my life, and when I developed MS, swimming became my #1 form of exercise. Three times a week, I have religiously gone in the pool to stretch, exercise, and practice things I had/have trouble doing on land (like standing, walking, and balancing). The water is cool and safe. It helps with spasticity, circulation, vascular, respiratory and digestive systems; it also burns calories and is a great de-stressor. On days when I'm not in the pool, I do a variety of exercises I have learned over the years from my dancing days, physical therapy, TV/videos, etc. I am still able to lie on my back and pull my knees up to my chest and rock from side to side, which feels "painfully good" for my severe back pain from spasticity. My goal is a 30-minute workout, but if I'm too fatigued, I'll give myself a vacation day from it. Throughout the day, I've learned to keep bending and stretching by trying continuously to do some light housekeeping. Again, I do what I can do, but when my body starts screaming "enough!" I quit, lie down and rest. If there is a period of time I can't do these things because of a relapse, for instance, my physical therapist has taught me gentle exercises I can do in my wheelchair for each part of my body (such as head/shoulder rolls, arm extensions...) Minimally, if I have no energy at all, my husband will stretch my legs and back for me, which helps my spasticity tremendously.

5. Don't get sick or physically hurt.

MS is an autoimmune disease. When a MSer gets sick or hurt, those fighter T-cells from our immune system get to work, but unfortunately goof up on the job and attack our nervous system instead of the real villains. That means inflammation in the nervous system will likely occur, causing present MS symptoms to worsen and possibly cause new symptoms to appear. Because the immune system isn't working properly, recovery time is lengthened for everything. So, I constantly wash my hands, don't share food or drinks, stay away from people with colds or viruses, keep my resistance up by doing #1 and #2 above, never put my fingers in my mouth, nose or eyes, and avoid situations that could cause falls. With regard to flu shots, I don't get them. (See Doctors/ Hospitals/

11

Vaccines chapter.) That is my own personal opinion. I choose to use commonsense methods to avoid the flu regardless of what doctors or researchers advise about shots. I've had a great record of not getting the flu all these years and don't want the risk of any side effects from annually developed vaccines on what the "new" strains are expected to be. In the event I would be in a situation that would require a tetanus shot, for example, I would consult with both my internist and neurologist about it.

6. Minimize stress.

Yeah, right, huh? Stress has been analyzed for years to determine if and how stress affects the body. I roll my eyes at these analyses. Personal experience and anyone with MS I've ever talked to *knows* stress has a direct impact on MS in the short or long term. All types of stress— physical, mental and emotional. Short-term stress will cause a worsening of systems from an hour up to a day or two. Getting three phone calls from solicitors in a single morning will frustrate me and cause me to drop things more, throw my legs into spasms, or prevent me from inserting a catheter into my bladder. (I've learned to take the phone off the hook at times.) Long-term chronic stress will cause a flare-up or full-blown exacerbation. One has to figure out his/her own way to combat stress. Swimming and exercise help me, or taking a time-out action such as getting on my scooter and taking the dog for a walk. I'll read, call a friend, shop on the internet, do yoga or lock myself in my room. Though I'm not a big user of anxiety or pain pills, I will sometimes take a Lorazepam and lie down if I'm emotionally drained. Somehow, waking up after a sleep puts me into a calmer state of mind. I'll go down my list of "bad-day" questions (see *Bad Days vs. Flare-ups* chapter) and take appropriate action if I can. I might just be hungry, hot, or thirsty. However, chronic stress is a whole different ballgame. Later in the book I'll share some of the major things in my life that caused chronic stress and how I managed it, sometimes alone and other times with professional help.

Finally, go ahead and **vent**! Most of the time (probably 90%) I do very well, but then that moment arrives. The shoe that took me five minutes to put on falls off. I drop a box of spaghetti on the floor. I have to pee so badly, but I can't get the catheter in. So, I scream, yell, cry, swear, or throw things. I give myself a break to let go and lose control. I try to direct my outbursts towards the sky and not at anybody, and then retreat to my room for a while to calm down.

7. Pace yourself/find support.

It took me years to learn how to do this. I was a perfectionist, a do-er, and was never a laid-back person who could let the dishes stack up in the sink. In the beginning, I was working full time and raising a family and just didn't understand how to put myself first and make the time to pace myself. After countless collapses, meltdowns, and spells where I was laid up to the point where I could barely walk, I started to learn what to do. I learned how to say "no", ask for help, hire help, accept help, delegate, take off work, go on disability, and do what so many people do when they have a cold or flu: lie down and rest/sleep. Get up, do a few priority things, then lie down and rest/sleep again. I have MS and that means I am sick. If I push myself too hard, I will get sicker. My doctors, therapists, good friends, peers and some family helped me with this enormous challenge.

8. Talk to a peer.

"I find discussions with other MSers to be more helpful, informative, enlightening and therapeutic than I could derive from any book or resource. Somehow, only those with MS know exactly what it feels like and how frustrating it can be." (My personal diary, January, 1986.) I can let my hair down when talking to a peer and not be pretentious. I keep in touch with some peers who are now precious friends that I met over 20 years ago. When we ask each other how we are doing, we can honestly answer back that we are lousy, or worse, or depressed. A very close friend of mine was dying of cancer nine years ago and would call me from time to time to talk. She said she was so sick and wiped out from the chemo, but family kept pushing her to get out of the house for some fresh air and diversion; that she shouldn't focus on the bad things. She would tell them to leave, then call me to pour her heart out and say, "I know you get it, and I need to talk about it." She was right; I did get it, even though I had

MS and not cancer. Fortunately, I have a few great friends that I can let my hair down with as well.

9. Ensure self-esteem.

As MS progresses, things become harder to do or some things just can't be done anymore. I was a dancer, but can't dance anymore. I was an active outdoors person, and can't hike, ski or ride a bike anymore. I loved sewing, but can't do needlework anymore. I gave up my career in banking and had to go on long-term disability. I would lose confidence, feel useless, and feel guilty that I couldn't keep up with things; depression would set in. I had to do something with myself, for myself and find ways to accomplish things differently to feel worthy. With therapy to help me with my negative feelings and jumpstart me, I used my imagination and brain to create new adjustments over these past decades. In the earlier years, I did volunteer work for the National MS Society and my son's school. I learned to speak Spanish and tutored kids for 15 years. Then I published a book and learned social media. I have been successful and generally happy.

10. Keep a positive attitude, faith and hope.

It's my nature to be an optimistic person. I look for the bright side of things, the silver lining, and believe there is usually a way to overcome obstacles. I believe with all my heart and soul that my positive "I can do this" attitude has enabled me to manage MS all these years. I ask for help and find support when I need an attitude adjustment caused by depression or feeling crappy. There are many times when hope seems hopeless and faith diminishes; it's a struggle to keep all that in check. If I am around negative people for too long, I remove myself and find a more positive setting. I have sadly seen some people go downhill quickly because of an unhealthy attitude. (See *The Optimist and the Pessimist* in Debbie's Favorite Blog Posts section at the end of this book.)

PART II

WHAT IS IMPORTANT TO KNOW?

Newly Diagnosed?

I've always believed that getting started with anything that you want to do is the hard part.

It doesn't matter whether it is starting a regular exercise regime, losing weight, quitting a bad habit or learning something new. Getting started with MS after you've received your diagnosis is no different; neither is the journey along the way.

Because of the unpredictable nature of the beastly MS, the types of symptoms, frequency and duration of relapses and resulting residual damage will constantly vary. New things will have to be learned, and the getting started over and over again is a given.

It's like pregnancy or parenthood. No one can prepare you for this. What your expectations were or what the real experience turned out to be is like night and day. But I will make these general statements from what I learned and how I manage:

- You have to experience and learn your own body. It will take time.

- Your first flare-up (or exacerbation, attack, or relapse) will usually be the most difficult and longest.

- Be careful about getting too many treatments prescribed at the same time, because it will be too confusing to know what is helping what.

- Keep a journal. You will start to see patterns and learn how your body acts and reacts. An easy way to do this is to use a 12-month calendar, with large blocks to jot brief notes in. It is helpful to see patterns when you are looking at a whole month at one time and easier to reference.

- The greatest fear is the unknown; so, become empowered by knowledge. I suggest starting with the National MS Society and other National MS Associations. (See *Resources/Bibliography* at the end of the book.) **But**--there is so much information and so many other resources available. It will become overwhelming, confusing and perhaps create more fear. Take baby steps when gathering information.

- Your best source of comfort and information will be from another who has MS, a peer. Be selective in who you talk with—talking with too many unknown bloggers can create conflicting opinions and confusion. Again, I suggest starting with your local chapter of the NMSS or other MS Associations for a trained peer counselor and/or interactive groups.

- Everybody has advice, what they've read or heard…use discretion and your own good judgment.

- What works for one may not work for another. If something doesn't work, try something else. Keep an open mind.

- You will need to find the best neurologist, PCP (primary care physician), and other professionals. But remember: doctors and other professionals aren't always right. Consult with them, but ultimately you have the last word.

- Back burner opinions (including your doctors) about the type of MS you have, or what the expected course/pace will be. There is no crystal ball and every case is different no matter what "the trends" are. Too often, these instill fear. Collect information about what's going on with you, like a scientist would.

- You are in charge of yourself. Do what you think is best for you and fits your personality. If you are in doubt about something, say "no." You can always reconsider later.

- You will need a lot of support, no matter how independent you are or want to be. You will need to get it from the right places. Support means both physical and emotional help, empathy (not sympathy), and assistance from your spouse /partner, family, health care professionals and friends.

- Staying healthy is essential. This is your immune system that is not working correctly. When you get sick, you will be twice as sick and it will take twice as long to recover. Relapses usually result in some residual (damage). It's a must to keep your resistance up—food, sleep, stress management…

- Exercise regularly. Start today.

- Accept and remember that this is a chronic illness. This is extremely difficult when you have to work, raise a family, and do the other thousands of daily demands. You will have to adjust your lifestyle. This change is slow and frustrating; it will try your patience and morale. But trust me, it can be done.

Here's an excerpt from my personal journal, December, 1985: "I hurt. I'm so tired. I feel like a mechanical robot breaking down. This disease really kicks it out of me. I really start dragging after lunch, then it's all downhill. I'm a real bitch. How do I keep on going? My body feels like it's fighting a virus day in, day out. Will I ever get a break? I don't know what to do." If you've read *My Ten Commandments* chapter, I now know what to do.

If you are newly diagnosed, you obviously have seen a neurologist. How was your experience? One of your top priorities in getting started is to make sure you have the best doctor(s), that you like them, and trust them. Take a look at the next chapter about doctors.

Note: Getting an MS diagnose is a difficult and often long process. (See *Diagnosing Multiple Sclerosis* in the Debbie's Favorite Blog Posts section at the end of this book.)

Doctors/Hospitals/Vaccines

---

*"I can't believe my doctor called me back on his cell phone,
just two hours after I called his office!"*
(My personal journal, April 2009)

<u>Doctors</u>

- You will need a neurologist, *one who treats many people with MS.*

- You will have a lifetime relationship with your neurologist and PCP, probably a urologist. Decide what you want from your doctor and what the relationship needs to be. Find doctors and professionals that *treat others with MS, and fit your personality.* Interview the office/doctor before you make your appointment. Ask yourself what you want/need from the doctor and the office, such as

  - good bedside manners
  - prompt responses
  - office visits
  - follow ups
  - experience
  - reviews

  I'll use myself as an example:

  I don't want a hand holder; I want someone I can *consult* with. I am not a whiner and when I call, that means I need help ASAP. I want called back that day, action within a day. I don't want to be dragged into the office when I'm too sick to get out

19

of bed. I don't want MRI's every year. When I go into the office, I don't want to wait an hour. I've got a fatigue problem. I want to talk to my doctor, not the receptionist. I want my doctor to be connected with the latest studies and research.

- Find a doctor in the top 10%. (My neurologist is a neurologist that other neurologists would go to.) Find a doctor who has many MS patients. Get referrals from: your local MS Society chapter, family, people you know in the health field, and other MSers. Check their background and credentials on the internet. Two websites I use are www.vitals.com and www.healthgrades.com, but there are others; you can do a Google search using a phrase like "doctor reviews and credentials" to get other websites.

- *You* are in charge, not the doctor. You hired the doctor, and if you are not getting satisfaction, fire him/her and get another one. My first neurologist (Dr. Pathetic) was a disaster. He was not informative, he didn't answer my questions, he didn't make eye contact with me, and he even had the audacity to use a dictating machine about another patient while looking over my file! My first neurologist when I moved to Phoenix was also a disappointment (Dr. Real Pathetic). I knew I was in a flareup and asked for Solu-Medrol. He insisted I was having a pseudo (false) exacerbation and wanted to double my antidepressants. I knew myself well enough to know what I needed after having 20 years of MS flare-ups. It wasn't more antidepressants. After he finally agreed to give me what I wanted, I walked out of his office forever.

- Go to the office or call on the phone prepared. Have your questions written down, have your problems written down with specifics. You will only have 15 minutes with your doctor, if that. Don't expect to be educated by the doctor. Expect answers to your questions. If you have a lot to talk about, schedule a longer appointment.

- Make sure all of your doctors share your reports and correspond with each other about your case, new drugs being prescribed or changed, etc.

20

- Realistically, the most your doctor will do for you is to prescribe medications for symptoms, encourage disease modifying treatments and make recommendations to other professionals. Don't allow yourself to feel pressured into anything you don't want to take.

- Will your doctor support you if you want to try some different alternative medicine? For example, in 1990 I had gone to Germany to try an MS treatment that was offered there but not approved in the US. My MS was progressing rapidly and the few experimental drugs that were under clinical study in the States were of no interest to me because of the potential risks. I did extensive research and decided I wanted to try it. My neurologist #2 (Dr. Excellent) supported me both before and after I went. He was my hero. And also, my neurologist for over 20 years.

- You need to feel that you trust your doctor.

Hospitals

Avoid them as much as you can, whether you are the patient or just visiting someone. They are unsanitary, full of infections, and make a lot of mistakes. An MSer can't afford to get an infection. However, there will be times when you will have to go to a hospital. Here are some tips:

- *If you are the visitor*—take hand sanitizer with you and use it often, such as in a bathroom, after reading magazines or shaking hands with someone. Keep a distance from people who show symptoms of a cold or virus. Avoid rubbing your eyes, sharing food, or putting things in your mouth, like a pen. Take your own bottle of water in lieu of drinking from a water fountain. Try to limit your stay.

- *If you are the patient*—use the same suggestions above, but also be extra alert to those who come in and out of your room. For example, is the nurse handing you medicine to take or the person giving you your food tray wearing gloves? Get out that sanitizer! If someone who wants to visit you is sick, suggest having a phone chat instead. Sometimes your doctor may want to admit you into the hospital to get Solu-Medrol treatment for a MS flare-up. Consult with him/her as to whether you can have the treatment at home. It's difficult to rest or sleep in a hospital since nurses frequently come and go to do things like monitor your temperature or blood pressure. By all means, *don't hesitate to ask someone for anything you may need*, like lowering the temperature if it's too hot, giving you an extra pillow if desired, etc. (See *How to Deal with People* chapter.) And believe it or not, too often the medical staff does not understand MS which is disheartening. The upside? At least they have heard of MS or know someone who has it. If you take the opportunity to become a not-in-your-face-educator, the nurses and aides are genuinely interested in learning about it.

Vaccines

What to know about Flu, Shingles, Pneumonia and Covid-19 Vaccines:

- People with MS may be at higher risk of getting shingles, the flu, etc. because of reduced immune system function from disease-modifying treatments. High-dose steroids, often used during relapses, may also increase the risk.

- People with MS can't receive vaccines that contain a live virus. It puts them at even greater risk of developing the very disease they are trying to protect themselves from.

- Since the Shingrix vaccine to prevent shingles does *not* contain a live virus, it is considered quite safe for people with depressed immune systems. Shingrix is recommended for folks over 50+ years. The occurrence of shingles is highest when you are older, sick, extremely stressed out, have a weak/depressed immune system. (e.g., from a physical injury, steroids, chemo, DMTs...) About one out of every three people in the United States (if they had chicken pox) will develop shingles in their lifetime. (Source: CDC) Being a senior, I know a lot of people who had shingles; *it is nasty*! My opinion? I'd take the shot over getting the virus.

- Vaccines that help protect against pneumonia work well, but cannot prevent all cases. On the other hand, although a pneumonia vaccine can't prevent all cases, it can possibly lesson the symptoms. Unlike seasonal flus, pneumonia often requires treatment in the hospital and can be deadly. The CDC recommends the vaccines for people who smoke, seniors over 65+ years and all people with certain medical conditions.

- The more people get vaccinated, the more other people can determine the probability of safety and effectiveness. The Covid-19 vaccine is a great example. Hundreds of millions of people have received the shots without severe, adverse effects. There is comfort in numbers. What is *not* known is how severe or deadly *your own* case would be if you got Covid-19. There are MS organizations like https://www.iconquerms.org/ collecting data specifically from and for MSers. I had the Pfizer shot with no severe side effects; I recommend it.

- Despite a belief that maximizing immune health will protect you, sometimes it just isn't enough protection. My opinion? Weigh your own risks according to *your* lifestyle, overall health, and age.

What to do?

- Consult with your neurologist about possibly adjusting the timing MS treatments so that vaccine effectiveness isn't lowered. And remember, you are immunocompromised if taking DMTs or steroids.

- If you choose not to get a vaccine, take commonsense measures to protect yourself. Wear a mask for protection against Covid-19, flu, and other viruses when around people to protect yourself against *them*. Friends and neighbors have commented to me that they experienced less sickness last winter, and will wear them again this winter. Why not? We have stylish masks in our drawers and are used to them. It's amazing to me how many people cough or sneeze without covering their mouth/throat. Yuk.

- Make a list of pros and cons for getting the vaccine. (See the *Making Decisions when Managing MS* chapter.)

An Ongoing Grieving Process

Most of us are familiar with the grieving process when a major event occurs in life (e.g., death, divorce...); a person goes through the steps of denial, anger, bargaining, depression, and acceptance.

A person with MS goes through this in the beginning with their diagnosis. For example:

Denial: "It can't be MS—I'll get a second opinion."
Anger: "Why me? "It isn't fair!"
Bargaining: "If only I didn't push so hard..."
Depression: "Just let me lay here and cry; I don't want to ever get up..."
Acceptance: "OK. Now that I know what it is, what can I do about it?"

As time goes on, a person with MS will have new symptoms that appear and old symptoms that worsen. Frequency and intensity will vary. It is grueling, scary and fatiguing. When will it end? Will it ever stabilize? How will it end? What residual damage will there be?

Each time there is a loss of function, the physical, mental, and emotional adjustments to lifestyle will have to be made. The grieving process will occur many times, over and over again—always different, never final. In the mind of a person with MS, one wonders, "when is the next time and then what will I have to deal with?"

Once in my early years, my husband in a moment of frustration said "Get used to it. You're not the only one with a walking problem and it can be a lot worse." Well, I did get used to it, but then it did get worse. And I had to get mad, go through the process and adjust all over again. It's like a roller coaster that you can never seem to get off of.

MS Symptoms—Overview

What are MS and its symptoms?
What did I learn and how do I manage?

Obviously, there are volumes of information on this subject, but here are the basics of how I explain what MS is:

MS is a disease of the central nervous system, an autoimmune and inflammatory disease. In a normal person, nerve cells in the brain and spinal cord communicate with each other by sending electrical signals down long fibers called axons, which are wrapped in an insulating substance called myelin.

In MS the ability of nerve cells in the brain and spinal cord to communicate and conduct signals to each other are affected. The body's own immune system attacks itself, causing inflammation and damaging the myelin. Myelin is the substance covering the nerve cells that enables the communication or nerve conduction. This process is referred to as demyelination. When myelin is lost, the axons can no longer effectively conduct signals. The result? Scars ("scleroses" is Greek for scarring) or better known as plaques or lesions in the brain and spinal cord, which is mainly composed of myelin.

MS takes several forms, with new symptoms occurring either in discrete attacks (relapsing forms) or slowly accumulating over time (progressive forms). Between attacks, symptoms may go away completely, but permanent neurological problems often occur, especially as the disease advances over the years.

- There is bad news and good news about MS symptoms.

First, the bad news: *almost any neurological symptom can appear with the disease, and often progresses to physical and some cognitive disability.* These include changes in sensation such as loss of sensitivity or tingling, pricking or numbness; muscle weakness, spasms, or difficulty in moving; difficulties with coordination and balance (ataxia); problems in speech or swallowing; visual problems; fatigue; acute or chronic pain; bladder, bowel, and sexual difficulties. Cognitive impairment of varying degrees and emotional symptoms of depression or unstable moods are also symptoms.

Now, the good news, and this is what one should focus on: *Not everybody gets all of these symptoms, and those that occur don't always happen at the same time. The prognosis over the long term for the majority of persons with MS is very good, especially with the exponential, recent growth in treatments, research and technology.*

- Symptoms that appear and hang around for a long time after a relapse could mysteriously disappear, or diminish. In my early years, I used to get optic neuritis often with my flare-ups. But, I don't anymore. The optic neuritis and its symptoms (See *Vision Problems* chapter.) always went away when the flare-up was over. I was bothered with cold feet sensations for many years, but haven't had this symptom in over ten years.

- If you think something is "not right" (feeling right, working right…), it probably isn't. You are not imagining it, and it's not in your head. My neurologist #2 told me this in one of my first visits with him, when I asked about the sensation of a bug that felt like it was crawling inside my forearm.

- Some symptoms will not go away after a flare-up (e.g., spasticity in one leg), may worsen temporarily if stress occurs (intensified spasticity in that leg) and then worsen with a subsequent flare-up (spasticity in both legs).

- The unpredictability of what symptoms may occur, how long they will last, how bad they will get, and if they will go away will be one of the most frustrating things you will have to learn to deal with. Everybody is different, and you will have to be the one to figure out these answers. I kept a detailed journal, and I started to learn the patterns of my symptoms and course of my MS after about five years. To this day, I still keep a journal.

- Many times, symptoms are a "chicken-or-the-egg" situation. For example, fatigue can worsen gait problems, or gait problems may worsen fatigue. Spasticity may worsen pain or vice versa. Taking it a step further, constipation could worsen gait problems, which then triggers excess fatigue and so forth. There is so much interplay between factors affecting MS symptoms and symptoms affecting other symptoms. It becomes confusing trying to figure out what's going on, where to start, and how to remedy it.

- From my experience with MSers, if the onset of MS has more motor disturbances than sensory and the age is younger (e.g., 20 years old as opposed to 50 years old), the prognosis will apt to be more disabling.

- All symptoms are troubling no matter how small one may judge them to be in comparison to others. When I facilitated my disability group for the National MS Society, some members felt they shouldn't complain about their numbness, ear- ringing, itching, tingling… because others were using canes or walkers. That is BS ("Bo-shee")! I couldn't stress enough that they *are* disabling: they distract, impair, and interfere with everyday activity too, and one has to learn how to live with them and manage them. I always used to ask: "Is it right that a paraplegic shouldn't complain, because of what a quadriplegic has to deal with?"

- Most symptoms can be managed and controlled in a variety of ways.

  - The sooner you learn how to deal with a symptom, the better.

- Contact the National MS Society for information, direction, and *hooking up with a peer*. The National MS Society website has good information on what MS is and its specific symptoms. It is very easy to read and understand. There are other MS associations like this, such as the Multiple Sclerosis Association of America and the Multiple Sclerosis Foundation. (See *Resource/Bibliography* at the end of the book.)
- Patience is learned and change will happen; but it is slow and not easy.

Many symptoms are temporarily worsened by many things one wouldn't necessarily think about. While definitely aggravating, they are not causing damage to your nervous system. My next two chapters, *The Heat Element* and *Bad Days vs. Flare-ups*, discuss this.

The Heat Element

Although heat will not cause a flare-up or attack,
heat definitely aggravates the nervous system
and will cause symptoms to intensify.

Heat slows down the conduction of nerve impulses in all people, but is particularly bothersome to folks with MS. When a person without MS gets out of a hot Jacuzzi or sauna, they move much more slowly. By comparison, a person with MS might not be able to walk or stand at all. Decades ago, one test used to diagnose a person with MS was to put them in a hot bath for a while and then see what happened!

Heat can be caused by weather (especially when there is humidity), fever, room temperature, over-activity, hot flashes, being in the sun too long, etc.

So, what to do?

Speed up the conduction of those nerve impulses by getting and/or staying cool. Ice packs are a favorite of mine; I put them behind my neck, my back, or rub them all over me. I carry them with me in a little six-pack cooler if I'm at an outing on a hot day. Taking a frozen plastic bottle of water in the car doubles as an ice pack and ice water at the same time. Cold ice water and showers are very effective in bringing body temperature down rapidly when overheated. One can go from not walking to walking in a matter of minutes. Air conditioning is a must. Some people use cooling vests. A small spray bottle filled with cold water and crushed ice can be helpful.

Getting cool and staying cool reduces fatigue and weakness and helps the mood because you feel better. One time I was in an amusement park and became extremely fatigued in the hot afternoon. I went to the air-conditioned infirmary for an hour and took a nap with ice packs. It rejuvenated me enough to enjoy myself the rest of the day. By the way, taking this action also relaxed my concerned companions

In my earlier years, I used to take a cold shower before going out somewhere. It increased my walking and endurance.

During my first appointment with Dr. Pathetic back in 1980, he told me to stay out of the sun. When I asked why, he said because it isn't good for me, and moved on to another subject. After I changed neurologists, I told Dr. Excellent this comment and asked why I should stay out of the sun. He just shook his head in disbelief. He explained that since MS is an inflammatory disease, there is of course inflammation occurring. In commonsense terms, he said that if you had bruised your ankle and it was inflamed, you would put ice on it—not heat! It wasn't the sun that was bad for me, it was the heat. *

I was angry at myself for being so naïve. I learned two lessons right away—the importance of gaining correct knowledge about MS, and the importance of a good doctor who understood MS.

Tip: I keep cut watermelon in the fridge during hot months. It cools down the body in the *inside*, is 90% water so it hydrates you, and is packed with nutrients. Frozen grapes are great, too.

https://www.youtube.com/channel/UCF3qgI2kmbkL2QHLIAEdmpg

*The sun, in fact, is actually good for you. Research has shown that it is beneficial since it provides Vitamin D, especially for a person with MS. (See *Vitamins/Supplements* chapter.)

Bad Days vs. Flare-ups
(Relapsing/Remitting Types of MS)

"What the heck is causing what?
How do I know what to do?"
(My personal journal, April, 1985)

"Bad Days" are what medical books and neurologists call pseudo exacerbations. I think this modern term can be very confusing because it is not an exacerbation at all (even though *pseudo* means false.) So, I'll just stick to the old-fashioned term we all used years ago, which has really the same meaning. *A bad day results in something that causes a <u>temporary</u> worsening of symptoms. No treatment is necessary, and there is no residual damage.*

- MS is very sensitive to so many things, such as
    - weather changes and types of weather (barometer, heat, humidity, storms)
    - sickness (colds, viruses…)
    - lack of food, water, sleep
    - medication
    - stress (temporary, not chronic)
- A bad day can last from several hours to a full day to perhaps several days, depending on the cause.

- There can be such wide variation in the severity of symptoms. Forgetting to eat could cause tingly hands, while having a bad argument could cause excessive fatigue or spasticity.

- Sometimes a bad day is the result of what I refer to as a "pay day." For example, if I wake up one day feeling great, I might push myself too hard to do extra things; then I "pay" for it the next day and can do only half of my normal daily activities.

- When you figure out what the culprit is, it can then be remedied and the symptoms will calm down. Heat can cause many things to go haywire. For example, in my early years I had a very high fever that actually paralyzed me. When I frantically called my doctor, he told me to crank down the a/c, lay in bed with ice packs, take aspirin and drink lots of water. When my body temperature came down, I could stand and walk again within a day and no residual effects.

- When the bad day(s) or spell is over, things go back to their normal state, whatever "normal" is to you.

"Flare-ups" (also known as exacerbations, attacks or relapses) *cause new symptoms and/or a worsening of existing symptoms that last for longer periods of time— weeks, or even months*. Personally, I like to use this term as opposed to the term "exacerbation" because it sounds less frightening.

- Resting often doesn't make a flare-up better. Treatments such as corticosteroids may be required to shorten the duration or severity of attack. (See *Treatments* chapter.) The MS is active, inflammation is occurring, and residual damage often results.

- A flare-up can just happen on its own, but often it will be triggered by any major physical, emotional, or mental stress, such as:
    - falls, accidents, sicknesses, infections;
    - *chronic* physical, mental or emotional fatigue or stress;
    - major life occurrences (death, divorce, new baby, abuse…).

Figuring out what is going on and what to do about it is frustrating and confusing. And there's always that "chicken-or-the-egg" question of trying to figure out what is causing what. Is my depression (fatigue, etc.) causing a bad day or flare-up, or is the bad day/flare-up causing the depression (or fatigue, etc.)???

To start, you can go through a checklist of things, asking yourself these questions:

For a possible "bad" or "pay" day, or ("spell"):
- Are you thirsty?
- Are you hot? cold?
- Did you sleep well?
- When was the last time you ate?
- Is it humid?
- Did you take your medication(s)?
- Did you start a new medication?
- Are you constipated?
- Did you rest?
- Did you overdo it?
- Do you have your menses? Are you in menopause?
- Do you have a cold? Infection?
- Did you recently fall and slightly hurt yourself?
- Did you just have an argument, or are you upset about something? Are you stressed and why?
- Are you sad? Frightened? Angry?
    - do you think these feelings will subside within a day or two?

For a possible "flare-up":
- Do you have any *new* symptoms or are existing symptoms intensified?
    - for how long? A day, days, weeks...?
    - how are the symptoms changed?
- Have you had any illness, colds, virus, flu, *any* type of infections?

- what, and how long, and how long ago?
- Did you recently fall? Hurt yourself?
- Have you been experiencing constant stress?
  - for how long?
  - why? (Work? Change with a job? Marital problems? Divorce? Death? New child?)
- Have you been in an accident, had any other physical injury?
  - how long ago?

What to do?

I make myself rest and give myself at least a week for the symptoms to calm down. Most of the time, they do. I try not to get on steroids too often, because of both the short and long-term side effects. (See *Treatments* chapter.)

If I have a cold, virus, or sickness, I try to hang in there and tolerate the MS symptoms until the sickness is over. Again, recovery from these for a MSer is usually longer because of our immune system dysfunction. The waiting can be a real burden on our patience, adding stress. I don't want to be too aggressive and get on steroids right away because steroids suppress the immune system, perhaps making recovery even longer. Prolonged, overuse of steroids is also not good for bone health. I'll take extra steps to rest, take care of myself, build my resistance up, and try to recover on my own. *If the cold/sickness is over and the MS symptoms stay intensified afterwards, then I call the doctor for steroids because at this point the MS is probably active.*

If I have an infection and can't treat it on my own (for example, a urinary tract infection), I call the doctor for an antibiotic. When the infection is gone but the MS symptoms are not going away after a week or so, I call my neurologist to discuss next steps.

If I have suffered some type of physical injury, I get treatment right away for the injury. Depending on the injury, I may also contact my neurologist for a joint consultation as to what to do. For example, years ago I slipped and tore my right rotator cuff. I went to my internist immediately to determine the extent of the injury and necessary treatment.

I was in severe pain, and I knew a flare-up was imminent. All my symptoms went haywire. When I called my neurologist, we decided going on the Solu-Medrel would be a prudent move in this case because of the injury, the inflammation, and the unfortunate fact that I now couldn't use three of my limbs. Both doctors communicated with each other; and treatment and physical therapy were arranged.

The next chapter outlines available treatments for MS.

Treatments

While there is still no cure for MS, there are options available to treat the symptoms and the course of the disease. But first, DO YOUR HOMEWORK!

To keep things simplified, there are three main groups of treatments, all with a different purpose: Medications, Corticosteroids, and Disease Modifying Treatments. In recent years, another group has emerged— Remyelination/Restoration.

<u>Medications</u>

These are used to treat the *symptoms* of MS, and the use can be short or long term. They minimize the intensity or effect of symptoms so the quality of life and daily function is more manageable. In Part III, I mention a number of meds that I use(d) for symptoms such as spasticity, bladder/bowel dysfunction, depression, sleep, anxiety… Most can be used safely for short or long-term use.

When a new symptom pops up and lingers on for a week or two, it's time to check with your neurologist and other sources to determine what may be available to try. I'll leave the specific medications up to you to find and try, but will make these general statements:

- **Start, stop or change only one medication at a time**. You will be able to better monitor the effects—both positive and negative—and decide if it's working or not. *It's bad judgement to be prescribed multiple prescriptions from multiple treatments at the* *same time.* In addition, many meds will take a week or two to kick in (an antidepressant for instance) so allow a couple of weeks for each change. Take notes detailing if, how, and what is improving.

- **I've said it before and I'll keep saying it: if one isn't working, consult with your doctor about a different dose or drug.** There are many meds available for the same symptom.

- **Weigh the benefits vs. the cost (i.e., side effects) of the medication.** All medications have side effects, including possible side effects from your other MS symptoms. If the medication is causing more negative side effects than the benefit you are getting from it, then stop it. *You* decide—don't be swayed by your doctor or somebody else if your gut tells you something is not right for you. When Avonex (a disease-modifying agent discussed a little later in this chapter) was first approved for MS in the 1990s, a woman in my MS group said she spent one or two days in bed with flu-type symptoms every week after she got the shot. After six months, she decided that the unproven percent of reduced relapses was not worth being so sick every week.

- **Research side effects of a medication on your own and read the inserts that come with the medication.** A doctor or a pharmacist will never tell you everything. While nobody will get all of possible side effects listed, it's worthy to be aware of them. For example, I take Ditropan for my bladder. A side effect of Ditropan is that I do not sweat. This can be very dangerous, as I will overheat very easily and living in the desert, I can get heatstroke. Another example is baclofen that I use for spasticity. If I take too high of a dose, it will cause my tight, spastic legs to become too weak.

- **Many side effects can be minimized or managed.** Since Ditropan works so well for me, I get around the not-sweating side effect by drinking a lot of ice water, always having an ice pack around, and avoiding heat. Ativan (for anxiety) will make me sleepy, more uncoordinated (dangerous for driving, walking or transfers), and my head fuzzy. So, when I take it, I try to rest. The benefit of less stress, anxiety, more rest and an elevated mood is worth the side effects. Calcium supplements are constipating, so I take two Tums daily to get my necessary calcium. (Note: An antacid will sometimes impact the effectiveness of a medication—check the inserted information page that comes with the medication.)

- **Research what contraindications the med can have with other meds you are taking.** Again, a doctor or pharmacist will probably not tell you everything, if at all. A huge example here is that if you are using a birth control pill, many meds will reduce the effectiveness of the pill and you may have to use an additional form of contraceptive to be on the safe side.

<u>Corticosteroids</u>

Corticosteroids ("steroids")—usually Solu-Medrol and prednisone-- are used to reduce the duration and severity of a flare-up (or exacerbation, or attack). Solu-Medrol is given intravenously for 3-5 days usually at home (about 1-2 hours per day). Prednisone is given orally usually over a 10-14-day period, beginning with a very high dosage (e.g., 80mg/day works for me) and tapering down the last week to 10 mg. by the last day.

There is much to know about steroids, and unfortunately, the doctor and the pharmacist never tell it all. The first experience with steroids is horrifying to say the least, and creates tremendous confusion and stress. I hated them in the beginning, but after I understood my own body's reactions and the fact that they did work for me, steroids became my friend.

What to know about steroids?

- The purpose of steroids is to reduce inflammation. Because the dosage is very high, the immune system will become suppressed. Therefore, you want to take all measures to keep your resistance up and your exposure to infections, colds and viruses low. If you currently have an infection or virus causing the flare-up, try to get rid of the infection/sickness before getting on the steroids if possible.

- A very common side effect of steroids is water retention. Eliminate as much salt as you can from your diet while taking them. This goes beyond table salt. Canned, frozen and packaged foods, pickles, condiments, luncheon meats, etc. are loaded with sodium; so, avoid these and eat bland and fresh foods.

- Appetite usually increases when taking steroids, so stick to snacks like carrot sticks, celery, almonds, apples, or unsalted popcorn. The sacrifice of a strict food regime for a maximum of two weeks is well worth the extra pounds you won't gain and have to worry about later.

- Once you start steroids, follow the complete program and do not just quit taking them. If you do, it can inhibit your adrenal glands from producing the natural amount of cortisol later.

- A universal complaint is insomnia. Speak with your doctor about sleeping pills. Even with a sleeping pill, you may only get four to six hours of sleep. Try to read, do paperwork, or anything that will keep you from dwelling on not sleeping. If you are anxious, consider asking your doctor about an anxiety pill to minimize stress.

- There are many other side effects when taking steroids; the amount, type, duration will be different for everyone. For example, I get supercharged and euphoric when I'm on steroids, especially when they kick in and my symptoms are improving. I also get very constipated.

- Try to temper your expectations and not compare yourself to anyone else. Some people respond faster and better than others. Take notes everyday about what is improving, what isn't, how much… It will help with your next episode. You will learn your own body reactions and patterns as time goes on.

- When a steroid program is finished, a person will often go into drug withdrawal. Symptoms may worsen again, and different side effects can pop up. For me, I get the shakes, anxiety, weepy, acne, some hair loss, sleepy; and my symptoms will be worse than before

I even got on the steroids. After my "withdrawal" period, my symptoms will adjust to what will be normal for me; and all of the other side effects from steroids will go away. After having been on steroids on average of twice a year over a lengthy course of my MS, I've learned what to expect and how to ride it out.

- Ninety to 95% of the time, a course of steroids will end a relapse. But some MSers can't tolerate the side effects. An alternative may be ACTH gel injections. ACTH promotes the natural production of steroids, but it is expensive. In the eighties, this was popular in shorting relapses and I was given these, with success and less side effects. This treatment had disappeared for years, but emerged again as a tool to lesson inflammation.

Note: Prolonged use of steroids can contribute to osteoporosis later in life. Staying on top of calcium levels is important.

Disease-Modifying Treatments (DMTs)

Disease-modifying treatments reduce the progression and activity of the disease. Most of them are for folks who have the relapsing-remitting form of MS, or for those who have secondary progressive disease and continue to have relapses.

Today there are almost two dozen FDA-approved DMTs available to treat MS. Research is ongoing to continue finding more. (Source: American Brain Foundation) All of them somewhat reduce the severity of relapses, the number of lesions; most seem to slow the rate of disability. Many DMTs have been developed in recent years, so data for these reductions continue to be collected and refined.

So, how is a DMT chosen?

Doctors will (or should!) first consider the severity of a person's MS. Risk factors of disease course will also be considered. These include things such as the person's age, sex, lifestyle, and other medical conditions. Finally, doctors will discuss things with an MSer like:

- How the DMT is given – oral meds? injections? IV infusion?
- DMT scheduling – at home? frequency?

- Plans for pregnancy – none? near term? long term?

As mentioned previously, it is difficult to predict a person's course of disease. That is why a newly diagnosed person is wise to keep a journal initially, and ongoing. Doctors will usually begin with a trial-and-error plan—their view usually is to consider the course to be long-term, but have a Plan B to switch the treatment if there is ongoing disease activity (i.e., relapse, new lesions).

- Most newly-diagnosed folks usually do not have a highly active case. So typically, a doctor will recommend one of the oral treatments or, less commonly, an injectable drug.

- A small amount of MSers (about 10%) have a very active course from the onset. So, a doctor will recommend a more potent DMT in the beginning. The thinking is that these will be more effective in reducing relapses, with a trade-off of more severe side effects.

- In recent years, there has been a trend toward a more aggressive treatment approach, including people with a less active disease. The reasoning is that increasing suppression of the immune system will reduce inflammation, thus reducing damage. However, in this situation, a person must consider the risk of having less immune function to ward off other potentially dangerous triggers like illnesses or chronic stress that compromise health.

- *DMTs (like steroids) cause the immune system to become suppressed. (i.e., "immunocompromised") Therefore, you want to take all measures to keep your resistance up and your exposure to infections, colds and viruses low.*

DMTs are a complicated decision, requiring collaboration between the doctor and the MSer. Personally, I believe that a newly-diagnosed patient should not be pressured or rushed in their decision. *The risk of taking a few months to think this through is no greater than the increase in potential disease damage.* Try steroids/other medications first. In my case, after the initial relapse subsided, I was absent of any new symptoms for a couple of years.

41

Important Tip: Make a list of all medications, including vitamins/supplements that you take (dosage, frequency, etc.), and all of your doctors' names and phone numbers. Carry this information with you in your wallet or purse, and give a copy of it to those who live with you or take care of you. You never know if you will have a medical emergency, be involved in an accident, etc. It happens. (Murphy's Law!)

Remyelination/Restoration

There is nothing yet to *stop* MS progression, repair the damage and restore function. But research and clinical trials are happening, and scientists are optimistic these could happen in the near future. It is also known that remyelination can occur spontaneously.

A wide range of areas are under study for demyelination/remyelination therapies—drugs, non-drug (how diet, exercise and gut microbiome affect the nervous system), and stem cells. Scientists continue to gain new insight into the risk factors and causes of MS, like gene research.

Stem cells are a popular subject many MSers inquire about. It's not surprising since the media/ads create a lot of buzz about the "amazing cures" for so many body ailments. In the MS arena, hematopoietic cell transplantation therapy (HSCT) is a new treatment that's currently being studied in the U.S. and other countries. Interest is growing in the field, and it's being evaluated in a few clinical trials. HSCT use adult stems taken from an MSer directly (bone marrow, fat tissue) and reintroduced later after the immune system is essentially eliminated with chemotherapy.

Other countries (not the U.S.) offer stem cell therapy for MS with a different approach. Basically, cord tissue-derived mesenchymal stem cells are used from full-term human umbilical cords. The cells are injected directly into the person via an IV infusion.

Bottom line? Stem cells offer great potential for repair and regeneration. Again, research is happening, but we're not there yet. It's a dangerous area—lots of hype, lots of risks. But there is hope down the road.

Are You Older?

"Celebrate your bigger birthdays. Age is wisdom and more memories." (Dr. Barry Hendin, M.D.)

The pace of everything I do has slowed. It is taking me longer to do things. Resting more each day is necessary. Motivation to go anywhere or do some things has dwindled. I can't exercise as long as I used to. There are many things I cannot do alone anymore and need help. Being a baby boomer, I have lots of company! Growing old is a fact of life.

When you grow older with MS

- **Immune health lowers as you age.** Bodies do not absorb vitamins and minerals as well.

- **Bone density weakens.** It's time for a bone density test. Prevent falls to prevent fractures.

- **Medications that you take have side effects.** Meds may cause more dizziness, fatigue, falls... Check out this article:

  More Elderly Take Drugs That Can Lead to Falls, (and more)
  https://www.yahoo.com/lifestyle/more-elderly-drugs-lead-falls-135551514.html

- **"Normal" people start experiencing many things that a person with MS may have been experiencing already:** leaky bladders, less balance and coordination, weakness, fatigue, less strength and endurance, cognitive issues. Aging is challenging enough, but aging with MS can compound many of these same problems. My fatigue and weakness escalated when I became post-menopausal. It's enough of a challenge for normal people but an extra challenge for MSers.

- **It becomes trickier to figure out what is causing what--is the MS acting up on its own, or is it re-acting to something else?** There is substantial interplay between physical, emotional, and mental health. Are cognitive problems a new symptom of MS, or is it due to aging?

I reached a point when I finally asked myself, why care about figuring out what is causing what? The focus now should be what can I *do* to help these things and prevent other aging issues. Like doing mental exercises and adjusting my exercise programs to maintain strength or endurance. Or, inquiring about certain vaccines and vitamins.

There are comments throughout this book regarding what to think about when older, like vaccines, vitamins, osteoporosis, cognitive function...

One more thing...

Whenever possible, strive to enjoy as many things as you can. But *you* decide ultimately what you want to do and if you can handle it. I've done a lot of amazing things so far in my lifetime, regardless of whether someone advised me to do it or not to do it. One never knows what the future holds or how fragile life can be. Having MS or another major issue will do that to you. You can't recover an opportunity after it is missed.

Other important things to address

This section starts out with a story.

About seven years ago, I called a good friend of mine whose husband died unexpectedly. She had MS over thirty years, was 70 years old at the time, and her hubby was her loving caretaker. We were MS buddies for 25 years, I checked in on her when all of the memorial activities ceased and the reality of her new situation began.

We talked about her present position and future plans. There are quite a few things I would like to share about our conversation that I believe are worthy to think about, for someone with or without MS. While these points seem practical, it amazes me how many people don't attend to them

- **It's essential to have a solid network of friends and family.** You just never know if your caregiver will pass or leave you. "J" is ambulatory, but she does have her limitations in other ways because of MS. J has no children. Though dependent on her husband whom she had a loving relationship with, she maintained her independence as much as possible. One of my favorite expressions is "Use your mouth and your intelligence", and J does that. Her wonderful circle of support helped her with the memorial and the aftermath of things to do, like her car and house.

- **It's important to have a plan in place in the event your caretaker/significant other leaves before you do.** Where would you live? Who could take care of what? Plans should involve short and long-term healthcare, short and long-term finances, wills, living wills, medical powers of attorney, memorial desires in writing. What do you want done with online sites? (i.e., social media, patient portals, etc.) *I actually started doing this after my son was born.*

- **Do you know where to find documents or how to do things your significant other does?** For example, my husband knows all about the "outside" of the house (e.g., circuit breakers, timers, sprinklers, all of info about our RV…) and I don't. I know all about the household finances, taxes, investments, insurance, where all the important documents are kept and he doesn't. We need to make the time to educate each other.

- **It is never too early to know how to take care of yourself and depend on yourself financially.** When my dad died, there were three of us kids (ages 20, 17, 9) and my mother (39) was a homemaker. I learned early to work, get a college education and into a high-paying career field, save and invest. Good thing. I got MS in my twenties. One never thinks it will happen to him/her.

- **Age is wisdom.** J and I talked about how well we know what is best for us and how we have the confidence to trust our intuition and judgment in making decisions. We also know when to reach out to a person we can trust to discuss something with. After all, two heads can be better than one.

- **Do what *you* believe is best for the present, as well as the future.**

I'm in the so-called Golden Years and retirement. It's time to let more things go and make the most of it.

P.S. "J" is currently well and happy, living in an independent apartment in a senior community. She's a 35-year MS survivor and is still ambulatory. She's been on DMT's since the nineties.

PART III

WHAT CAN YOU DO?

The Invisible Symptoms
"You look so good!"

---

*This phrase has irked persons with MS
for as long as I can remember.*

That's because on the outside so many of us *do* look good unless we have some kind of walking aid to indicate otherwise. We're not bleeding, we have good color in our faces, we're not coughing or blowing our noses. When we look good, people automatically think that we *are* good.

But we're not because so many of the symptoms are invisible. Pain, tingling, numbness, fatigue, dizziness, tightness, depression, blurry vision, balance, coordination—the list is enormous. "No, we are *not* drunk!"—say many MSers who hold onto walls or furniture to keep their balance. These symptoms interfere with everything we think, say or do. They are annoying; they hurt; they are frustrating; and they make us crabby.

Invisible symptoms are difficult to describe, and when we tell someone about them it's hard for them to understand or empathize. When we see these same people again, they forget that we have these symptoms because they are invisible. If we talk about them, we sound like complainers. Or, many times they are uncomfortable and don't know what to say. This was a topic of discussion in almost every disability group meeting I had. Peer-to-peer, we understood it, shared our stories, and how we coped.

A common complaint is something called "an MS hug". It feels like a tight band that squeezes you around the middle of your body. I can't stand to wear tight clothing.

When I was into my fifth year of MS, my walking endurance was limited to less than thirty minutes. If I pulled into a handicapped parking space, I was yelled at and given dirty looks. Amazingly, when I started using a cane later that year, people would stare at me when I pulled into a space but then quickly look the other way when I would get out and start hobbling slowly with my cane.

These symptoms are disabling. As my MS progressed, I've lost other abilities. Yeah, I hate it, but I had to learn to live with it, cry, and vent from time to time.

But the unpredictability of MS can give good surprises. About ten years ago, a newer friend of mine was asking about MS. It was obvious that I was disabled because I was in a wheelchair. But when I started talking about the problems with invisible symptoms, I used my hands as an example. My hands *looked* normal, but I couldn't:

- button buttons (I used a button-assist device)
- distinguish coins or other things when I put my hands in my purse
- type with all ten fingers
- hold a regular pen (I used only certain types with grippers)
- shuffle or deal cards
- tighten my grip, and often dropped things

Today I can do all these things! Was it remyelination that took place? Was it something else? I still don't know for sure, but it doesn't matter because they work again!

Fatigue-
A Different Kind of Tired

"People look at me and just cannot
understand why I get so tired."
(An MSer comment, March 2011)

Out of all the symptoms I and others have experienced with MS over all these years, I truly believe this is the one symptom that is the most difficult one for everyone involved. It is a universal complaint by over 90% of MS victims. For the 90% of us MSers, it is the "F" word!

It doesn't matter if the case is mild or advanced. It doesn't matter whether it's one of the relapsing/remitting or progressive types of MS. It doesn't matter if you had a good night sleep or if your MS is not currently active. Fatigue is always present with MS, 24/7. Why? <u>Fatigue exists because MS is a disease, a chronic illness</u>.

- You will get fatigued easily, whether other symptoms are present or not. Simple activities like making dinner or talking on the phone too long can exhaust you. The slightest thing can make it worse, such as not eating, drinking enough fluids, or being overheated.

- Your fatigue will worsen as the day progresses.

- Fatigue causes forgetfulness, lack of interest and little energy.

- Fatigue is compounding and escalates quickly if MS becomes active due to a relapse, or the amount of disability has increased over time. For example, sleep disturbances due to bladder problems at night, or extra effort required to walk because of spasticity or other gait problems will all impact fatigue significantly. Energy is reduced, weakness increases. This causes stress, frustration, and depression that will then lead to even greater fatigue.

- Fatigue is often caused by medications taken for other MS symptoms and bowel or gut disturbances.

Unfortunately, fatigue is extremely difficult for a non-MSer to understand. You can't really see it. Someone may say "you look tired, maybe you should take a nap." A nap may help, but fatigue isn't due to just being overworked or sleepy. I describe it sometimes like when you have a virus; when you feel so run down and wiped out all you want to do is lie down. Or, I'll give an example by saying that when trying to walk, each leg feels like it has a ten-lb. weight strapped to it.

So, what can be done about fatigue?

- **Rest frequently**. I lie down 1-2x/day for at least a half an hour, especially in the afternoon. In the years I was still walking but had gait and spasticity problems, I found ways to sit/lay to do things— using a stool in the kitchen to cook/iron, folding laundry on the couch, laying on the floor to play games and read with my son, and so forth. Learn to rest *before* reaching that point of total exhaustion.

- **Pace activities**. I do physical activities intermittently and limit the number I do in one day. For example, I do one load of laundry at a time. If I tutor kids on a Tuesday morning for a couple of hours, I don't plan any other outing that day. If I do a 45-minute workout in the pool, I limit my exercise program to mild stretching the next day. If I am going out for dinner, I rest and take a cool shower before I go. Learning how to rest frequently and pace myself was a huge life adjustment for me, but as my MS progressed, I learned to change my ways and accept the fact that I could no longer be superwoman. Truthfully, it took me years to learn.

- **Use the time of day you have the most energy for the most difficult tasks.** I am a morning person and that is when I feel the best and think most clearly. I'll do my physical activities like swimming every other day. On the days in between, I'll do my mental work first and then do low energy activities like dusting, later.

- **Ask for help/accept offers for help.** Obviously, resting more and pacing activities affect what can be accomplished. My habit of making a daily to-do list would start out with ten things, but I could only complete half of them. It caused a lot of anxiety as I was always such a doer, a perfectionist, a neat freak. My Aunt Dorothy was a caregiver for my son, and took him many times to give me a break, especially when I had relapses. For a while, we were able to have cleaning services. I had good friends that would vacuum or cook for me, or send their older kids over to do housekeeping. I learned to say "yes" to people who wanted to help.

- **Learn to say "no."** Personally, this was difficult for me, since by nature I try to please everyone. If I had to miss my son's soccer game or decline an invitation for a family gathering, I felt guilty. Over the years, however, the fatigue and increased disability forced me to start saying "no"; I just couldn't do it all anymore. As I mentioned earlier in this book, getting started is the hard part. Once I started to say no to things, it became easier.

- **Research or inquire about medications.** There are medications that are available that help *reduce* fatigue. They may or may not work for everyone, and of course if a medication is causing more side effects than benefits, then don't take it. For years I took Symmetrel (or the generic, amantadine) and it helped me enough to stay on it. A side benefit of this particular drug is that it is an anti-viral medication as well, so I would get a script from October through April during the virus seasons. Since it caused insomnia for me, I took it only in the morning. Likewise, there are medications that *cause* fatigue. For example, I take my antidepressant after my first bathroom trip during the night—it helps me fall back to sleep.

- **Consider using walking aids, devices, and other gadgets.** walkers, wheelchairs, canes, sticks, grabbers, stair glides, hand controls...I have or had them all, starting in 1984. They are essential to helping reduce fatigue and they work. What's good for me is also good for those around me. Trust me. (See *Let's Talk Walking Aids* chapter.)

- **Learn stress management tools.** Stress is a huge culprit in intensifying fatigue, and techniques such as relaxation, breathing, and visualization are incredibly effective in managing fatigue.

- **Exercise has been shown to benefit fatigue.** Listen to your body, though. Over doing it will wipe out the benefit and ruin the rest of your day. Icing for 15 minutes after exercising helps prevent fatigue.

Vision Problems

---

*Vision disturbances are often the first sign
of MS that ultimately will lead a patient
to a neurologist and an MS diagnosis.*

While the onset of vision problems is frightening to say the least, the good news is that most of these symptoms are not usually permanent.

Optic Neuritis

Most people who experience optic neuritis have MS. Usually one eye is affected, but both can be involved.

Optic neuritis is the primary cause of vision symptoms and includes blurry vision, partial or total loss of sight in usually one eye, spots or blind spots in the field of vision, dimness or loss of contrast in sight, and pain. The optic nerve is located behind the retina of the eye, and becomes inflamed, thus causing the problems. Swelling and slight discoloration of the optic nerve can be seen during examination.

Your neurologist will know if you have optic neuritis by looking into the eye. If your neurologist is the first to detect it, there's no need to go to an ophthalmologist and have a million tests done. This is because if you see an ophthalmologist first, he/she will ultimately refer you to see a neurologist anyway. My neurologist had given me a visual evoked response test in his office. The test results will show if the conduction of nerves is at a reduced rate, a sign that demyelination is present.

Optic neuritis can happen very quickly, sometimes within a matter of hours or a day. Generally, corticosteroids are used to reduce the inflammation and lesson the severity and duration of symptoms. Once treatment is started, the symptoms and inflammation usually go away within a week. Symptoms generally do not last and rarely is there permanent loss of vision.

Other Vision Problems

There are two other types of eye problems that can occur, but these are associated with brain stem and cerebellar attacks and not the optic nerves. The first is eye muscle jerking, or nystagmus, which causes vision to be "jumpy" or moving. The second type is eye muscle weakness, which can cause double vision. Double vision is often remedied by steroids or intermittent resting of the eyes.

Internal Plumbing
Part I: Bladder

The bad news is that almost everyone who is diagnosed with MS will develop bladder problems. The good news is that it can be successfully managed and you will be able to control it.

Bladder dysfunction occurs due to lesions in the spinal cord. Simply put, there is one of three problems.

1. Failure of the bladder to hold the urine. (The bladder is "spastic.")
2. Failure of the bladder to empty the urine. (The sphincter muscle that releases the urine is spastic and won't open.)
3. The combination of both 1 and 2 above.

The primary symptoms are:

- frequent urge to urinate
- frequent urination
- hesitancy in starting urination
- difficulty in keeping the urine flowing, or finish voiding
- incontinence
- nocturia—frequent voiding at night, at times without waking

The medical term for this is neurogenic bladder.

Obviously, this is a sensitive area for someone to talk about. At least nowadays, there are numerous and frequent ads and TV commercials that talk about bladder leakage. And there are so many protective pads and garments available today to prevent public embarrassment. However, when these symptoms start, you need to do more than just put on a protective pad and tolerate it. *You need to see a urologist who knows about MS and neurogenic bladders well, and begin to learn about bladder management as soon as possible.* Untreated bladder dysfunction can cause damage to the urinary tract, urinary tract infections (UTI's), or damage to the kidneys.

Now that I have nearly scared you to death, let me assure you that bladder management is easy to learn and do. Since my bladder problems started when MS was still in the dark ages, I didn't learn what to do for over three years. Today, that is inexcusable. I found an excellent urologist, who put me through several tests to examine and evaluate my bladder (dys)function. This is common practice. Then he taught me what to do and it changed my social and physical life immensely.

I am really proficient at bladder management and though the damage to my bladder function is severe, I have been able to be like a normal person, and nobody would ever guess that I had problems in this area unless I told them.

What to do?

- Again, start by finding a good urologist who knows MS. Through medications and other techniques, you will learn how to void normally: once every four to six hours.

- There are many effective medications available that will:
  - relax the sphincter muscle when you can't begin to void.
  - reduce bladder spasms so that your bladder can hold urine like a normal person and not leak.
  - promote urine flow.

  You can take a combination of meds if you have more than one bladder problem. There are many effective meds you can take for long periods of time. (I've been taking Ditropan to "hold the urine," and baclofen to "relax the sphincter" for thirty-five years.) You will learn how to adjust them if you need a stronger or weaker dosage. Adjustments may also need to be made with medications from time to time as your MS progresses or if you have a flare-up.

- Intermittent self-catherization, either for a limited time period or always. People would cringe in my MS groups when this subject came up, but after showing the slim, plastic 6" catheter and demonstrating what to do, the fear went away. It's easier for women than men, since women only have to insert it about one inch to get to the bladder. It's great for me when I'm in a place where there are no bathroom facilities because I can pee in a cup or bottle just like a guy!

  Tips: If you don't have insurance to cover the cost of disposable catheters, you can reuse the ones you have by always washing them completely with soap and water after each use and storing them in a plastic case or bag. Always start with clean hands and wipe your privates well before insertion. When the urine is flowing out, concentrate on pushing your abdominal muscles down. When the urine stops, try twisting the catheter a little to the left and right, as more urine might come out. Finally, when urine flow stops, exhale while you remove the catheter, otherwise you will get air in your bladder.

- Do everything possible to make sure your bladder is as empty as possible when you void. This must be done to prevent urinary tract infections. If you are sitting on the toilet and feel like you still have to urinate more, try a technique called Credé. Make a fist and push downward on your bladder six or seven times as you lean forward. Or while bending over, grab your arms together under your legs and bear down and push. Also, relaxation breathing works for some people.

- Many times, a residual of just three or four ounces of urine left in the bladder can lead to a UTI. To help prevent this, I take 500 mg. of vitamin C daily to keep the acidity level of the urine high. Many resources will tell you to drink cranberry juice, but I prefer not to drink the extra calories since vitamin C accomplishes the same thing. Do NOT eat or drink oranges or other citric fruits for *this* purpose as these actually increase the alkalinity of the bladder!

- Consult with your doctor about taking a daily antibiotic for your urinary tract as a UTI preventive if you self-Cath, such as nitrofurantoin or Hiprex. If it begins to become ineffective, there are others.

- Always drink plenty of water. (I do admit though that I refrain from water two hours before leaving the house for an outing to unfamiliar places since I don't want to be bothered looking for a bathroom—let alone a clean one.) If you don't self-Cath, refrain from drinking fluids two hours before bedtime. If you lay on your tummy for 20-30 minutes before retiring for the night, this also will help empty the bladder. You can tell by the color of your urine if you are drinking enough water. A dark color indicates you are not drinking enough—the color should be very light or clear.

- Be prepared for an accident or possible leakage if you are having a "bad day" or a flare-up. These will cause bladder symptoms to intensify just like any other MS symptom.

Urinary Tract Infections (UTI's)

If any of the signs below appear, call your doctor immediately and have your urine checked. A UTI will definitely affect your other MS symptoms as this is an infection, and if left untreated too long, will cause a flare-up and possible further complications.

- cloudy urine
- odor to the urine
- blood in the urine
- burning sensation with or without urinating
- urgency, frequency of urination—even if you are on medications to treat your bladder symptoms
- fever
- increased spasticity

If bladder problems do develop, then the bowels are probably also affected. Read on...

Internal Plumbing
Part II: Bowels

———————

This is another one of those symptoms that most MSers
have to deal with, and it's no fun.

When I used to have my group meetings, it was a frequent subject that everyone needed to talk about, and humor rarely was interjected as we talked. It interferes, it hurts or is uncomfortable, it affects our moods and it often controls our lives. We hate those people who get up every morning, and five minutes after having coffee are flying into the bathroom. We're sick of listening to how products like yogurt will make everything perfect.

It's either too much one way (diarrhea/ or can't "hold it") or not enough the other (constipation). Constipation is usually what we have to deal with, but when we finally explode and don't make it to the bathroom in time, it's humiliating. Too often there are many factors involved that cause our tricks and techniques to fly out the window.

There is much written on this subject as to how to manage it, and plenty of advice as to what to do—drink plenty of water, eat lots of fiber, exercise, take this, take that, do this, do that, blah blah blah. So yeah, we do all those things to try to keep our stool soft and promote regularity, but sometimes it all seems in vain.

Personally, I've had bowel problems since I was twenty. I have a lot of residual damage in my lower spinal cord that continues to progress over the years.

The medical term for this is neurogenic bowel.

So, what have I learned and what do I do?

- I follow all the basic rules for good digestion: lots of water, fruits and veggies, fiber, etc. to keep my stool soft, and exercise. But eating too much fiber can cause excess gas, water absorption and actually worsen bowel elimination so each person has to determine what is a good balance for themselves. i.e., I'm not "normal."

- I can't digest dairy products, which is probably good since they generally cause gas, bloating or constipation. I take acidophilus daily for "good" bacteria; calcium and vitamin D for bones and calcium absorption. (See *Vitamins/Supplements/Diet* chapter.)

- Get a referral for a gastroenterologist (GI) doctor who understands neurogenic bowels *as they relate to MS*. Not all of them do.

- I don't listen to people who say you have to have a bowel movement every day. My GI has reassured me that I *don't* have to go every day, especially if the colon has been completely emptied by natural or other means.

- My GI also told me years ago that if I don't go after two or three days, I need to take steps to make myself go. If I feel that my feces are way down by my anus, I insert warm water from an old Fleet bottle, or use a Fleet. My sphincter muscles are weak and often need a little stimulation. This works for me. Some people use suppositories successfully for this reason; again, you have to try different things and do what works for you.

- Every other night I take a product called Perdiem (the kind in the *yellow* plastic bottle) that contain sennosides. I have been using these for years, a recommendation made by my first GI. They are gentle with no cramping and work well to keep me rather regular. These can be bought in a pharmacy or online. I have also had a lot of success with a product called ColonMax. It's a natural laxative made with herbs and magnesium hydroxide for occasional constipation. Sometimes I need to take one a night for a couple of days, but I have no cramping or hard stool when elimination occurs. There are all types of products like these on the pharmacy shelf or online that can be tried. If one doesn't work, try something else. GI doctors have an arsenal of meds to try and keep you regular.

- Again, if after that third day, I feel like the stool is more upper colon than lower, I take Miralax, a stronger laxative, or a full enema. This is necessary, and a good gastroenterologist knowing MS will agree to this. Don't get worried about the "laxative dependency" warnings that labels or people will tell you about regular laxative usage. We have MS and must do this. Finally, don't get worried if the label says results will happen the next day and it doesn't; sometimes it takes two or three days. Every digestive system works differently. And, we aren't "normal". (Note: The comments in this section were confirmed by several gastroenterologists that I have seen over the years that work with MS patients.)

- When I've done all of the above and don't have a BM after a week, (not often), I go to a *licensed* practitioner and get a colonic (hydrotherapy). Medical doctors frown on this, but it's natural, safe and usually provides immediate relief. Eastern medicine has been doing this for years; the Egyptians did this 4,000 years ago; and many quads and paraplegics do this. Just don't get sucked into going every week—that's not necessary. Occasional use is best. If you are not comfortable with this, then it's definitely time to consult with your doctor.

- Once, after 16 days of not having a BM, my doctor sent me to the ER. The bowels were impacted--I was foolish to wait this long. They prescribed a liquid substance to drink that finally started to give me relief. The interesting thing is that I was full of *loose* waste. So why wasn't I going? The normal contractions in the colon/sphincters that push the waste through were not working because of my MS nerve damage... I did get completely cleaned out, and after a couple weeks of a daily laxative regime the gastroenterologist put me on, my colon started to contract and function again.

- When I go through spells when my colon becomes overactive, I have a few tips.

  - I blow out short breaths constantly until I get to the toilet. It's an old Lamaze trick I learned when pregnant: when you blow out, you can't bear down and push. However, you have to really concentrate.

  - I have an extra set of panties, clothes, wipes, plastic bags packed for my car, or anywhere else where I might be. Back in the eighties I had an "accident" at the office and fortunately had a bag packed in the back of my desk drawer.

  - I keep a bed pad between my mattress and sheet, and in my car.

  - Since I have a 'script for Hiprex because I self-Cath, I double the meds on days I lose my bowel control so that I don't get a urinary tract infection.

  - I cheat. If I really have to go out somewhere, but am afraid of having an accident, I don't eat or drink anything until I get home.

- Many medications will affect your bowels—steroids, antidepressants, bladder, and especially pain medication. They will usually constipate you. Drink extra water to stay hydrated.

- Bowel problems will cause fatigue, stress, and aggravate symptoms. My spasticity and back pain always worsen when I'm constipated.

- When I need to vent or talk, an MS peer is always the best choice. "Normal" people don't really understand the bowel implications due to MS. They do more talking than listening with their advice, and sometimes say things that are scary. No—I won't need abdominal surgery if I don't have a bowel movement for a week.

- Finally, I remind myself to relax. I'm not alone, and I *always* eventually go!

Keep reading to understand a bit of another subject that has emerged involving digestion…

Internal Plumbing
Part III: The Gut

"More crap--as if things aren't complicated enough trying to get my plumbing to cooperate. This is helping to explain everything that's been going on with me over the last year."
(*My personal journal, January, 2021*)

Our health and our gut (stomach and digestive tract) are tightly linked to many aspects of physical and mental health--digestion, mood, brain, heart, and immune function. The gut houses 70% of the cells that make up the immune system, so keeping the gut healthy and balanced is critical.

Good and bad bacteria live in and on the human body, mostly in the gut. When they are out of balance, it's known as *dysbiosis.* Dysbiosis in the digestive tract can cause gaps in the barrier walls around the digestive tract allowing the bacteria to "leak" into the bloodstream. Studies have shown that dysbiosis could be a cause or an effect of MS. Thus, a variety of digestive symptoms are caused.

These are the main complaints, but the list could include many other physical, mental or emotional disruptions:

- Bloating, gas, cramps
- Aches and Pain—abdominal, back, head, other
- Constipation, diarrhea
- Nausea
- Food sensitivities, loss of appetite

- Enhanced MS symptoms, such as more spasticity, neuropathy, fatigue...
- Moodiness, anxiety, stress
- Skin disorders

What to do?

Unfortunately, the complications of MS become more complicated. It's a tricky business trying to figure out what is causing what. The leaky gut problem aggravates the MS symptoms and vice versa. Or are these symptoms just a result of the neurogenic bowel or IBS? It's disheartening, frustrating and exhausting. I was in tears more often than I would care to admit before I starting understanding everything.

When I began telling my different doctors about how awful I was doing, they all approached it from their area of expertise. Even my gastroenterologist began with treating my neurogenic bowel and IBS. Not one of my doctors mentioned dysbiosis, or leaky gut. After a year of different tests, trying different meds one-by-one, monitoring my foods, I started to research it on my own. A friend had told me about dysbiosis, the affect it had on her life, and why.

My own life had been affected due to a severe head concussion and prolonged, chronic stress. I started a recommended probiotic. Finding out about this leaky gut stuff was a relief. These are the main areas to focus on to keep your gut healthy and balanced:

- **Get quality sleep**. Studies have that shown poor, (or lack of) sleep disrupts microflora in the gut, lowering immune health.

- **Reduce stress levels**. Long term, constant stress has devastating effects on gut health which cause serious gastrointestinal conditions.

- *Tip:* Try peppermint essential oil. Not only is it soothing, it contains antispasmodic properties, which can relax the muscles in the digestive tract. This can help relieve constipation. I dab it on my wrists.

- **Add a probiotic supplement to your diet**. Probiotics disrupt the overgrowth of toxins/bad bacteria and prevent them from passing through the intestinal lining into the bloodstream, where they wreak havoc and cause illnesses.

- **Make healthy food choices**. A Mediterranean diet is a good place to start. Note: While a lot of fiber and fresh veggies are always recommended for good digestion, one's own body can be sensitive to many foods, much like lactose intolerance. For instance, I discovered too much fiber was as disruptive to me as too little fiber; I could tolerate steamed veggies better than raw ones. Too much sugar caused discomfort.

If you are following the above four bullets, don't assume gut health is the cause of your crazy MS symptoms; it is worthwhile to just be aware of it. But, if you are highly suspect that this may the reason you are experiencing persistent digestive issues, you could inquire about a microbiome test. This identifies specific bacterial and fungal species and compares *your* gut to a normal gut microbiome. Lab results help identify if/how to improve gut health.

While talking about these things that involve areas below the waist and between the legs, let's now move on to another one of them: sexual dysfunction...

Sexual Dysfunction

Sexual dysfunction is a complicated and distressing symptom of MS, with 70-90% of persons with MS experiencing this problem.

It's a fact: the central nervous system (CNS) damages the nerves fibers that enable sexual arousal, feelings and function. The damage happens the same way as it does to cause other MS symptoms. The prevalence is high like bladder and bowel impairment, since many of the same nerve axons or tracts are affected.

Adding to direct effect of the CNS, the MS-caused symptoms like fatigue, spasticity, and emotional disturbances further compound the sexual issues. All of this can result in (but is not limited to):

- decreased or no genital sensations
- decreased or no sex drive
- difficulty in obtaining an erection or orgasm
- decreased lubrication
- decreased muscle tone

Needless to say, the impact on a person's life and self-esteem as well as the life of the couple is enormous and can be devastating.

What to do?

I'll be blunt. Communicate, experiment, be open-minded. Just like "normal" people, sexual issues are complex and everyone's pleasures and needs are different. There are a variety of therapies and professional counseling that can help treat both physiological and psychological sexual problems. Sometimes, things can't be treated.

First, one has to acknowledge and accept the fact that there *is* a sexual problem and a real reason for it. You can't pretend it doesn't exist, or you and/or your relationship will spiral downwards rapidly from the emotional stress.

Then, communicate, communicate, communicate—with your partner, with your doctors, with your closest MS peers. You need to get out into the open what problems are occurring and search for ways to solve them. Any therapy should involve both partners; be open-minded and experiment to both of your comfort levels. If your partner isn't willing to go to therapy with you, then go to therapy yourself so you learn how to deal with this part of your life. It's too important to ignore.

Spasticity, Ataxia, and Weakness

There are many symptoms affecting the normal use of our limbs in MS that are caused by the damaged myelin in the brain stem, cerebellum and spinal cord. Though the spectrum of symptoms is wide and frightening, it should always be remembered that not everyone will get all of them, and many will be mild. For the mild symptoms that progress to a more advanced degree, they really are manageable.

These symptoms more often affect the legs more than the arms, hands, and other body parts and generally will start off on one side of the body. Thus, it is the problems with gait that most people tend to associate and identify with MS and seem to be most concerned about--the fear of ending up in a wheelchair. Forty years ago, the popular statistic was that 25% of people did end up in a wheelchair. But again, with the new treatments and therapies available, I would assume that this number is much lower nowadays.

Unfortunately for me, I had to deal with a variety of gait problems from my very first flare-up in 1980, and the problems mounted quickly. I will share some of this a bit later, but first I will explain the most common symptoms. Most problems can be helped to some extent by physical therapy (including exercises and gait training), the use of appropriate assistive devices and, in some cases, medications.

Spasticity

Spasticity is an increase in muscle tone, which really means that the muscles do not relax as much or as easily as they should—they actually contract. Because of this, spasticity affects movement and is considered a "motor" disturbance. Severe forms of spasticity can cause walking to become difficult, then subsequently causes fatigue and posture problems to follow. When the doctor checks knee or elbow reflexes, they jerk quickly and are much exaggerated.

Spasticity causes a limb, usually a leg, to stiffen and cause the joint to lock, or jerk; or the limb can contract and cause the leg to bend inward; the limb can go into spasms, or produce a feeling of tightness, like you have thick rubber bands or duct tape strapped around your legs or even your trunk. Another problem from spasticity is clonus. Clonus is when muscles jerk or twitch repeatedly. The most common form of clonus is when a person's foot taps rapidly and repetitively on the floor, or when a knee or ankle jerks repeatedly. Spasticity also can occur in the lower back, causing feelings of tightness or even pain in the back.

What to do?

Don't panic, and don't just live with it. I have had severe spasticity for years and have it managed so well that people don't even know I have a problem with it. If my foot starts to tap rapidly, I simply bend over and do some deep breathing while I stretch my back. The tapping stops within seconds.

When spasticity starts to appear, find a good physical therapist (who knows MS) through referral or contact your local MS Society Chapter to learn stretching exercises and other exercises to stay limber and flexible. To this day, I can still touch the big toe of a straight leg to my nose.

Try learning yoga, breathing and relaxation techniques. The more you move and bend and stretch during the day, every day, the better off you will be. Talk to your neurologist about medications specifically used for spasticity such as baclofen. These are generally effective in treating this symptom with minor side effects. Some people say that cannabis helps.

Spasticity intensifies easily to things like heat/humidity, constipation, stress or even lack of water. Other triggers include anxiety, fever, pain, bad posture and infections. Take care to prevent these factors as much as possible or be aware of them. As time goes on, you will begin to note and remedy them. You will be surprised at how quickly you can reduce spasticity as quickly as it increases.

Finally, spasticity can work to one's advantage when legs are weak. For instance, I use a power chair all the time, but because of the spasticity in both legs, the stiffness enables me to stand. I practice doing this throughout the day. With the ability to stand, I'm able to be more independent, dress myself, use a small bathroom, and get out of my car into my chair more easily. In addition, I have osteoporosis, and the weight bearing exercise of standing is very good for this condition.

Note: Many people say that cannabis helps reduce spasticity. However, when using cannabis, be careful if you take medication for spasticity because your legs may weaken too much and buckle.

Ataxia

Ataxia is a common symptom of MS, and is usually the result of lesions in the cerebellum. The cerebellum is the lower part of brain responsible for coordination of movement and balance. Problems can involve walking, rising to a standing position, swaying to one side like one is drunk, clumsiness and lack of coordination when using the legs, and/or using the arms and hands together, or jerked movements with tremor.

What to do?

Begin with balance exercises, like standing on one leg especially with your eyes closed. Visualization can help. I was taught years ago to imagine that my feet were in a foot of concrete. It worked for me—I used to practice this, standing in front of a sink.

The core, or trunk of your body is the foundation of your balance and stability. There are beneficial exercises to strengthen abdominal, back and pelvic muscles. Incorporate exercises in your daily routine. When I walk my dog with my scooter, I try to see how far I can go without leaning on the armrest. Fifty-lb. Grizzly tugs a lot.

Yoga is effective in improving balance and strength, with additional benefits of improving flexibility and fatigue.

When starting these different exercises, they will probably seem hard to do. Start slowly and gradually increase the activities. Remember, getting started is the hardest part. Google away, or hook up with a fitness trainer or physical therapist. Many exercises can be done at home; you don't have to go to a gym. At home, you can spread your exercises throughout the day.

> *Tip:* MS Exercises for Balance (MS Fitness Challenge)
> https://www.youtube.com/watch?v=d2tUxMlr5zA

People with severe ataxia generally benefit from the use of assistive devices, like canes or walkers. (Read the next two chapters about walking aids.)

Weakness

Muscle weakness is a common cause of gait difficulty and can cause problems such as toe drag, foot drop, compensatory hip hike, trunk lean, or swinging a leg out to the side. Weakness can also be caused by damaged nerve pathways in the spinal cord, and can occur in one or both legs. Though more prominent in the legs, weakness also affects the arms and hands. For example, coordination and fine movements of the hands (ataxia) can make writing, combing one's hair, and tying shoe laces very difficult. It can also affect tremor, where the limb or limbs shake, or possibly vertigo or dizziness (along with nausea).

What to do?

Weakness can often be compensated for with the use of strengthening and other appropriate exercises, starting with what I said above in the previous section. I keep a strengthening ball handy and practice gripping and squeezing when I'm on the phone or watching TV. I do the same with barbells and resistance bands. Again, assistive devices help and many are available.

Tips: If you have hands that are weak or have trouble gripping, Swedish dish cloths are great. I love them since I can easily wring the water out with one hand. Check them out on Amazon.

Let's talk walking aids...

---

*There is still a stigma about using walking aids.
People feel "funny" using them, or they may feel that
they are "giving into" the disease.*

As I mentioned, I had gait problems from the very beginning of my MS. By the time my son was a year old in 1984, I was 29 and could only walk— I had lost the ability to skip, hop, run or dance. I started using a cane at the age of 30. By the time he was four, the weakness and ataxia had progressed to the point I could walk only a maximum of thirty minutes before collapsing, and constantly had to hold onto walls, furniture, handrails to walk or climb steps. At that point, I bought an electric scooter for part-time use—I was only 33 years old. Four years later in 1992, I chose to use a walker full-time. The walker enabled me to walk further and better, improved my posture and reducing back and shoulder strain. My MS was frequently active and very aggressive.

I never hesitated to use any assistive device and actually sought them out on my own and here's why:

- I chose to play it safe. I didn't want to fall and injure myself, and risk more flare-ups and residual damage. Years ago, I accidently tore my right rotator cuff and that old injury is haunting me now.

- I wanted to keep active, live life with more ease, and enjoy my family. I could have never gone to the zoos, amusement parks, Disneyworld, shopping malls and so many other places if I didn't have my electric scooter.

- Assistive devices allowed me to be less fatigued, which elevated my moods and enabled me to do more. I didn't overheat as fast since I struggled less in trying to walk. Since I was walking better using the devises, I experienced less muscle and bone stress on my body parts.

- People—family and strangers alike—treated me differently. I *looked* disabled and received many more offers for help.

- What helps you, helps others! Seriously.....

..... using walking was the best choice for me *and* my husband. I would never have had the stamina, energy, ability to travel extensively and accomplish the endless things in my life. There was less pain, frustration doing things in a power chair; enhanced my quality of life. Doing things that were easier and less painful to me was also easier and less painful for my husband, or anyone with me. I was able to be more independent—then and now. I don't need to have anyone with me 24/7.

I get angry when walking aids are portrayed or perceived in a negative, fearful way. **Let's face it—when the term "multiple sclerosis" is mentioned, the initial thought is the "wheelchair." And the fear of using one. Gr-r-r! Get fearless!**

Fortunately, the attitude and awareness about using medical devises has changed since the eighties when I first had to use them. People of all ages are often seen in movies and advertising brochures using a wheelchair. You see more people out and about using them. For example, grocery stores, stores like Walmart and Target have electric scooters available for people to use in their stores while shopping. Many places like amusement parks rent wheelchairs and scooters.

When I got my 3-wheel electric scooter in 1987, many people looked at me quizzically. I actually was asked many times from older people, pregnant women, and others who wanted to know where to get them, how they worked, and how much they cost. I used to buy canes in different colors and styles to match my outfits. When I bought my walker on wheels, complete with handbrakes, a seat and a basket, the product I bought came from Sweden. No one had seen such a walker before—so practical and functional, with a seat to rest on and a huge basket to carry things around for me. Now, you see them *everywhere*! It's so gratifying to see such acceptance, and it really is helpful when someone has to take that first step to use one.

As a group leader, I often encouraged folks to think about eyeglasses. Why? We buy them to help us see better and don't think twice about it!

*Tip:*If you are timid or self-conscious about using a walking aid, try one out in a discreet location. You may ask a physical therapist how to use a cane or walker, for example, then borrow one and try it at home. Or, you can go to a medical supply store and with their assistance, ride around the store and parking lot. Once you experience how much benefit you get from a walking aid, you will have more confidence. Remember what I mentioned earlier about getting started!

A note about excursions and travel:

National and state parks are ADA compliant, as are most public places now throughout the U.S. My husband and I visited all 50 states, Canada, Mexico, seven countries in Europe, and the Caribbean. **Most of these trips I made in a wheelchair. Truthfully, I could *never* have done it without one.** Planes, trains, buses, cruises and steamboats. I was lifted into helicopters and a hot-air balloon that had a seat. My scooter was disassembled and put in the 7-seater plane when we flew into Nantucket. We found most places had accessible accommodations like hotels, museums, etc. People we met along the way were extraordinarily helpful. One time when I wanted to eat in a restaurant on the second floor of an old, inaccessible building, four guys insisted on carrying me in my chair up the steps! All you need is a mouth and a brain.

(See *The Truth about MS and Wheelchairs* in Debbie's Favorite Blog Posts section at the end of this book.)

Note*:* To get a handicapped or license plate, contact the motor vehicle department in your state for qualifications and forms.

Durable Medical Equipment

I asked for help, I wanted help, and needed help. I used my mouth and my brain to figure out what was out there and how I could get it. I put my research skills to use and found myself on a fast-learning curve.

I am an independent person. I like to do things on my own as much as possible, but I'm not too proud to ask for assistance or use a devise that will get me to where I want to go and do what I want to do. I wanted quality to my life and I needed to keep myself as safe as possible from getting hurt.

The types and varieties of assistive devices are endless, but again, you do have to do your homework to get the product that is exactly right for you. Buying an electric scooter today is as complicated as buying a car, and a salesperson is out to make a quick sale. Insurance doesn't cover many things and when it comes to durable medical equipment, the products sadly are way over-priced.

Go to medical supply stores to "window shop", talk to other people with MS, physical therapists who work with persons with MS, and surf the internet to look at different products. But do not buy something unless you try it out, and for the larger ticket items, get a trial period with a return after so many days if it is not working for you.

Let me give you examples of some of my experiences.

- When I bought my new GM station wagon back in the 90's, American car companies were offering $1,000 towards any handicapped device that was necessary. I got a lift to lift my scooter in and out of the car.

- It is very difficult to get approval by an insurance company or Medicare for a scooter. They don't view this as navigable as an electric wheelchair (also referred to as a power chair) in a house; and they don't care about fulfilling your special needs outside of the house. When I bought my last scooter, I found the exact one that I wanted, and then proceeded to buy it over the internet at a much lower price than a medical supply house. (It was $2,000 less than the local medical supply store wanted to sell it to me for.) I had to pay out-of-pocket for it because I get my power chairs through Medicare and they will only buy one wheelchair every five years.

- Make sure you figure out exactly how you will be using the equipment and buy accordingly. I use my scooter outdoors over grass, over gravel, going to the grocery store, going camping, etc. Thus, I made sure it was sturdy, had larger tires with good treads on them, a cloth seat (I stick to leather and it gets hot), etc. It has two 12-volt gel batteries and when they are fully charged, will go a distance of eighteen miles; this is a wonderful feature for longer excursions to places like parks or shopping malls.

- Even though I have an electric wheelchair for use in the house and a scooter for outside the house, I have a manual wheelchair also. I bought a small, light-weight one so if I am driving alone to a place such as a friend's house or restaurant, it is easy for my friends to put them in and out of the car. (I still drive my old station wagon and didn't invest in an accessible van yet.) Besides, a small manual wheelchair can often navigate house bathrooms and doorways much better than a scooter.

- Sadly, things like stair glides are not covered by insurance. In my old house in Pittsburgh, I needed two of them. I bought them used and my handy husband installed them.

- Many things like stair glides, lifts, and hand controls that are not covered by insurance can be bought secondhand on sites such as Craig's list. Also, contact places such your National MS Society chapter as a possible resource for these items.

- Hand controls for cars are extremely easy to learn to use. I love being able to drive my car—there are so many drive-through places. In addition, since I don't yet have an accessible vehicle, many times I'll go to a store like Target, call customer service, and they'll bring one of their electric scooters (or "carts") to me. Sometimes, I have someone load up my scooter in the back of my station wagon, go to the shopping mall and have a security guard unload it for me. Other times, like I did with Best Buy, I'll call a local store for something I want (for example, the pool store), explain my special needs situation and ask if they will bring it to my car. Most small, independent stores are accommodating.

  <u>Note</u>: *Check with the Motor Vehicle Department of your state to find out what you need to do in order to drive with hand controls. Generally, a prescription is required from a rehabilitation specialist.*

- Almost everything today can be rented or borrowed. I have rented cars with hand controls. Wheelchairs and scooters can be rented for a day's outing, or for travel to another city. Organizations have loan closets and only request a donation. When I flew to Denver to visit my brother for a week some years ago, I took my walker on the plane with me, and he had the loaned scooter in his home waiting for me so I could use it when we went for walks or other excursions. When I flew into Phoenix before moving here, I borrowed a manual wheelchair from St. Vincent DePaul.

- If you travel with your electric scooter as I have done countless times, you can drive it up to the door of the plane, then transfer to an aisle wheelchair while they load the scooter down in the belly of the plane. (Note: Make sure your battery type is acceptable on a plane.)

- Contact your local MS Association chapter for ideas, help, leads and financial assistance. Years ago, when I was a member in Pennsylvania, I received financial assistance from them for durable medical equipment.

- If your insurance company won't cover something that you feel should be covered, fight like hell! When I moved to Arizona, I bought a home with a built-in pool so that I could swim regularly to keep up with my aquatic therapy. I submitted my $2,300 receipt for a hydraulic pool lift. They rejected me. I appealed three times. During the final appeal, I had personal representation by the MS Society, my parents, and supporting documentation from my neurologist justifying the benefits of aquatic therapy for my symptoms, edema, respiratory and cardio-vascular systems, weight and overall health. I argued that $2,300 was the equivalent of only 12 physical therapy sessions. They finally approved me!

Pain

Through reading, experimenting and therapy I learned that there are many things that can give pain relief. I am still learning. I tried medical marijuana for the first time in 2011. I was desperate and thought, why not?

Pain is usually not a common symptom in the early stages of MS (except optic neuritis), but as the progression of the disease occurs it becomes a larger issue due to a variety of things.

- stress/tension
- spasticity
- posture
- stressed body parts
- nerve damage

In the beginning, I couldn't understand why things like aspirin or Bengay didn't give me relief. As my MS started to advance, pain started interfering with my life physically and emotionally. It depressed me and made me so agitated I couldn't concentrate on anything or be civil to people.

Here's a list of ways you can get relief for different types of pain and its causes.

- physical therapy
- hand-held massager
- trigger point therapy/massage
- yoga/deep breathing

- tai chi/Pilates
- exercise—swim/floor/balance and *frequent stretching*
- acupuncture/acupressure
- reflexology
- medication
- professional pain management programs
- medical marijuana
- soaking in a tepid, epsom salt bath

And, there are pain medications like Vicodin or Percocet available. I personally choose not to go this route since narcotics are addicting, cause constipation, and mess up my head and mental clarity. In recent years, opioids have become heavily scrutinized since they are potentially addicting.

Fortunately, many of these are recognized as effective pain relievers and are sometimes covered by medical insurance. I have tried most of them and have become very good at knowing which to use to reduce my pain. Try them—they work for many people! I've never had to enter a professional pain management program yet although these are beneficial to some folks.

Optic Neuritis

The pain behind the eye from an inflamed optic nerve can be excruciating. It can come on fast, even in a matter of hours, and is usually the start of a flareup. The first thing I do is put an ice pack on the eye for pain relief, which often works. The second thing I do is call the doctor for steroids ASAP. Steroids kick in pretty fast and usually will reduce the pain and any other eye symptoms one may be having from the optic neuritis since steroids are given to reduce inflammation.

Stress/Tension

Shoulders and neck muscles tighten, and jaws get clenched. Then a headache starts to develop, and the tightness/spasms from spasticity begin to intensify. The rolling stone starts gathering moss—fatigue and emotional stress are triggered.

What to do?

Relaxation is key for this type of pain. How do you know if you are relaxed? My physical therapist taught me this trick: Look to see if your shoulders are raised and your hands are into fists. Take a deep breath, exhale quickly and drop your shoulders like a shrug. Feel the difference and focus on the relaxed state of the neck and shoulders; your hands will no longer be fists. This is your goal.

If stress is from a temporary, emotional issue (like trying to get an insurance issue resolved on the phone,) I'll try to relax by using yoga and deep breathing, or vent to get rid of the initial steam. If that doesn't do it or if it's from overworking or emotional overload, I'll take an anxiety pill and lie down for a while.

If I get up and still have some pain, I'll exercise and work on my state of mind by listening to music, reading… Even though the pain is definitely physical, the mind set does matter. How you think about it does affect how well you manage it—if you focus on the bad, how much it hurts, etc., you may hurt worse.

Spasticity

As explained earlier, spasticity occurs when the muscles contract, tighten, stiffen, or go into uncontrollable jerky movements. It doesn't take much to the intensify the symptom so much as to cause pain from a muscle so tight or contracted that it "freezes" and is difficult to move. Muscle or joint pain is usually in the legs, but can also be in the arms, hands, and lower back.

What to do?

There are basically three things to help spasticity. The first is to try one of the medications available that specifically targets the central nervous system to reduce the contractions and tightness. I have taken baclofen, a popular med to help remedy this, for the last 37 years. It has always helped me, and as the years went by, I've had to increase the daily dosage from 20 mg/day to 60 mg/day. (I take 10 mg. tablet every four hours.) The most common side effect is drowsiness, but I don't really have much of this and it doesn't interfere with my daily activities. I have never tried the other meds available for this (such as Valium or Zanaflex) since baclofen has always been very effective for me and I tolerate it so well.

Another very essential thing to do is stretch all of your muscles *every day*. Make it a part of your daily regime like brushing your teeth. Spasticity can cause your muscles to contract up to an inch in a day, and daily stretching will help keep them in check. An experienced peer or a physical therapist can teach you how to do this. When the spasticity intensifies to the point of pain—stop, bend and stretch. If I get too rigid or fatigued and need help, my husband knows how to stretch my limbs and back for me.

Finally, learn and do breathing and relaxation techniques. Deep breathing and slow exhaling help spasticity. These tools reduce stress, which intensifies spasticity.

Stressed Body Parts/Posture

People like me who have (had) trouble walking will get pain from the additional stress placed on muscles, bones, tendons in trying to walk. Posture is out of whack, and as we desperately hang onto those canes and walkers, we use our upper body and arms more to pull along those heavy, dragging legs and keep our balance. It doesn't take long for those muscles to tighten, spasm, and really hurt. Even if in an advanced case of MS where one sits in a wheelchair for extended periods on time, there is a lot of strain on the back muscles just from sitting. Again, the rolling stone gathers moss—fatigue, spasticity and emotional stress soar.

What to do?

Learn and practice resting and pacing as much as possible. Massages give temporary relief. Trigger-point therapy, which I always describe as "feeling painfully good", is very effective in reducing my neck, back, and shoulder pain. When I couldn't afford to get massages/trigger point therapy (most insurance companies didn't cover these), my husband learned how to do it. He digs his thumbs down deep into the tightened muscle spasm to loosen up the muscle. Hand-held massagers can be quite effective. Sometimes ice packs help the inflammation, but sometimes heat wraps help soothe the pain. Experiment with it—if one doesn't work, try the other.

Go to a physical therapist (P/T) to learn how to work on balance, use walking aids properly, get the muscles stretched, and learn strengthening and muscles exercises. Make sure you find a physical therapist that knows MS and has experience with persons with MS. As my own MS progressed, I had to go for P/T a number of times to restore function and lost strength from a relapse. Or, to retrain the brain (yes, this is possible) to use different methods for balance, coordination and gait to compensate function lost due to the lesions. Techniques such as tai chi work both as a preventative and restorative for balance and coordination problems.

I found a physical therapist years ago who came to my home to evaluate how I stand, transfer, pee, get in/out of bed… She had over 20 years of experience working with MSers and was able to make sure I was doing things most effectively and safely. Since I had been using a wheelchair permanently over ten years, she showed me techniques to strengthen my trunk so that I could correct my leaning to the left side. She watched me do my floor and pool exercises and showed me ways to further enhance the effectiveness of what I was doing or could do.

My arms take a beating and often I get tendinitis in my elbows. Cortisone shots, arm stretches, and arm supports help to relieve the pain.

For many years I used a device called a *Swing Machine* and swear by its benefits. The machine is a square box about seven inches high with stirrups, that plugs into an electrical outlet. Lying on my back, I put my ankles into the stirrups and set the timer (which is included) for twenty minutes. The machine swings the legs side-to-side in a rocking motion providing relaxation, reducing stress and relieving back pain. It also increases circulation in the legs and feet and for me, reduces the swelling in my feet. I practice deep breathing and arm stretching while I'm in it. There is no stress on the spine or other body parts. My machine originally came from Japan (a gift from my sister); the basis of is to maintain a proper "chi" balance and positive forms in the body, an Asian technique. They are not very well known in the U.S. but I have seen them on the internet for about $150. Just Google *swing machine*; you can find and take a look at them online. Or, pull up my video demonstration. https://www.youtube.com/watch?v=KdrcJUrYHVs

Nerve Damage

Pain is transmitted by nerves, but pain from nerve damage is different. It doesn't originate from muscles or bones, but from the central nervous system as nerve pathways are damaged by the MS lesions. This pain has been described as burning, aching, or stabbing. Sometimes there are prickly or itching sensations. Sometimes sensations get "mixed up", where pain can be caused by your clothing. *Peripheral neuropathy* is the all-encompassing term for the malfunctioning of nerves due to them being damaged or destroyed.

What to do?

Forget anything over-the-counter and call your neurologist for a medication. There are certain medications that work specifically on nerves. I tried Lyrica and although it didn't work for me, it works for others. My old peer-friend Cathy suffered from severe pain on one side of her face. She took Tegretol, (considered an anti-convulsant) that was effective in reducing the discomfort. There are a number of different kinds available that one can try to see if/what works the best. I use ice packs on my lower back to numb the burning. Sometimes they work, sometimes they don't.

It was the "burning to the bone" and "knives in my back" pain that provoked me to call my friend and see if marijuana would help. I was amazed how it took the edge off and gave me relief. After a few trials I quit because I didn't like the effects it had on my mental state. The popularity of cannabis is increasing but here are some things to be aware of:

- There is ongoing study and debate about physical/psychological effects. These include memory problems, impaired judgement, slowed reaction time, weakened immune system, effects on digestion and respiratory systems. This is obviously important for walking and driving.

- In addition to short-term effects, there may be long-long term effects depending on how you take it, how much you use, and how often you use it.

- Cannabis can be expensive, and it isn't covered by insurance. It's also still not legal in many states.

When I try all of the tricks in my arsenal and nothings seems to work, I take a sleeping pill and go to bed. I want to knock myself out and get into deep sleep that will help relax my body.

Tomorrow's another day to take care of anything else.

Pregnancy, Menses and Hormones

"All three of these affect MS in some way. It's no wonder why women are three times more likely to get MS than men."
(My personal journal, 1992)

The first time I had finally read something about hormones having an effect on MS was thirty years ago. The article was in the September 1993 issue of *Scientific American* magazine. Today, there are all kinds of information and studies written on these subjects.

I mentioned in the beginning of this book that I worked a number of years in my professional jobs doing financial analyses and market research. One of the things I know from that experience is that conclusions of studies can be misleading by how the numbers are presented. I've become quite the cynic about this. For example, one might read "according this study, 50% of patients using XYZ showed a 38% reduction in…" What if the study only included ten people?

So, find out how many people were used in the study, what were their characteristics, how long did they take XYZ, what were their side effects, who did the study, etc. You have to dig deeper, be cautious, use common sense and talk to your professionals when you hear something of interest and want to pursue it (like having a baby or trying a new medication).

Therefore, I will address these subjects from my own experience, and those with MS I've talked with throughout the years.

Pregnancy

When I was pregnant 39 years ago, my MS was in remission and stabilized. I had a wonderful pregnancy and delivery. A couple of months later, I had a huge attack that went on for months. Was it caused by the physical trauma to my body? hormone adjustments? emotional stress? fatigue and lack of sleep from caring for a newborn? or, the added stress of returning to work seven weeks after delivery? Probably all of them.

I was left with a lot of residual damage. When I was teaching my son to walk at the age of one, I was losing my ability to walk. As I mentioned earlier, at 28 years of age, I could no longer hop, skip, dance, run, or stand on one foot. I got a cane for my 30th birthday for leg weakness and poor balance.

Does this happen to everybody? No! Many women who shared their stories generally did have a great pregnancy. And not all of them had flare-ups afterwards. I talked to a number of women who had two, three and four children that went through it all with flying colors. On the other hand, many women did suffer relapses after delivery. It is like a game of roulette. Some win and some lose.

What should one do?

- It's a personal decision and all the numbers in the world from studies can't tell you if *you* will be the one who will relapse or not. You have to weigh the cost of risk vs. benefit. For all the trouble I had after having my son, I would do it all over again.

- You have to consider what medications/treatments you are taking, and the risks associated with continuing to take them or not during your pregnancy. If you are taking DMT's, talk to your neurologist about your plans for getting pregnant.

- If you decide *not* to have children, be careful of the contraindications that *any* medication you take will have the birth control pill you are taking, even if it's an antibiotic or prednisone. Many doctors/pharmacists will not tell you this.

- You will need a lot of help and support, especially if the MS decides to become active. How strong is your marriage? No matter how good kids are, they are demanding and require as much energy in their teen years as in their toddler years.

- While this sounds insensitive, children are expensive, and may be an important consideration for you and your significant other. I'm being realistic and practical—MS can also be expensive due to medications, walking aids, loss of income, and so forth.

I desperately wanted a second child. When I discussed this with Dr. Excellent, he gave me a very practical answer to ponder. *"It's not the aftermath of the pregnancy and delivery I'd worry about—it's the next eighteen years of raising that child I'd worry about."* It hit me like a ton of bricks. I was struggling trying to raise one child. I had only my aunt who helped me with my son; I had little help from my husband during the work week or any other family member. My aunt was my son's caretaker when I worked, and took him overnight and on weekends when I was sick or needed to rest. She told me she could help me with one child, but couldn't with two. I knew I couldn't do it without her help; and, if I risked greater disability, how could I enjoy and cope with my kids as they grew up?

Don't worry about your children inheriting MS. While it is known that there is a genetic component that predisposes or makes a person more susceptible to get MS, it is not congenital (directly inherited).

Menses and Hormones

Most women with MS I've spoken with will have a slight temporary worsening of their symptoms the days before their menses start. Don't look for them, but if they worsen, it's not your imagination. They will go away, and no, your MS won't worsen in the long term because of them.

Birth control pills eliminate the monthly fluctuations of hormones for a lot of women. Less bleeding is less fatigue. Less bloating may occur. For those in their thirties and forties, they can minimize night sweats and hot flashes, minimizing the MS side effects due to the internal heat they generate. They can be helpful for the mood swings. I took birth control pills for years, and was better on them than off them. I took the pills continuously without the one-week break so that I wouldn't get a period at all. Since I do self-Cath to pee, it's less messy and risky for UTI's.

Again, what works for one may not work for another. You can try birth control pills to see if they work for you. If they cause more problems than the monthly, temporary worsening of MS symptoms, then they are not for you.

Hormones in any phase of a woman's life cause havoc, especially emotional issues. It doesn't matter what age you are or what stage in life you are in. Much to my chagrin, I still have night sweats in my post-menopausal age.

Emotions, Depression, Cognitive Functions

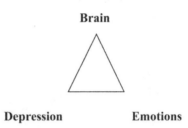

Brain

Depression   **Emotions**

Let's make a list of things that can cause depression or wide range of emotions that we can have (i.e., mood swings, crying, anxiety…).

- stress
- pain
- fatigue
- medications/steroids
- hormones
- frustrations with symptoms
- fear of the unknown

Could there possibly be more? Unfortunately, yes. *The brain itself.* There are areas within the brain that control our emotions, depression and even certain types of cognitive functioning that can be scarred with lesions from demyelination, *directly* causing these symptoms.

Talk about confusion! Stress can cause anxiety, moodiness and after awhile depression that can aggravate symptoms. Walking difficulties can cause depression that can cause emotional crying spells that can cause symptoms to worsen. Chronic fatigue and stress for extended periods of time can cause a flare-up that can cause inflammation and disease activity anywhere in our brain or spinal column.

How in the world can you figure out what's causing what so you know what to do? Is it the MS causing this or something else?

First, you can go down the "bad days" check list (see *Bad Days vs. Flare-ups chapter*) to see if you can identify what can be making you emotionally crazy or down in the dumps. Just by identifying what it could be can make you feel better or reduce some fear–maybe you are having your menses or are trying a new medication. Then take steps to remedy the situation to make you feel better. Maybe a cool shower will help, or taking the phone off the hook and lying down, or venting to a good friend... Whatever it takes for you to calm yourself down, do it. For me, complaining to a good friend willing to listen may not solve my problems, but it sure feels good to vent and cry on somebody's shoulder. When you feel better you do better, and your moods improve.

Now depression can be a bit trickier. It's one thing to be down in the dumps for a few hours or a few days. It's another to be depressed for several weeks or months, with constant feelings of sadness, lethargy, hopelessness, no appetite, lack of concentration or motivation to get out of bed. This is clinical depression and *must* be treated. It is *extremely* common in MS, and is very treatable. It's nothing to be ashamed of, because your brain has been affected by the MS.

Antidepressant medications will effectively treat the hormone imbalance that has been caused and perhaps some initial psychotherapy will help as well. I have been on Prozac for years, and a few times when I experimented and tried to go off of it, I discovered I needed it. I've been on it for well over 30 years, and I will always be on it. The only side effect I have is that it makes me sleepy, so I take it at night. There are many antidepressants available to try.

Cognitive Functions

MS can affect cognitive functioning to some degree but not severe enough to interfere with everyday activities for most people. The types of functions that can be affected are short-term memory, attention, concentration, or processing information. Long-term memory, intellectual, comprehension, reading and conversation skills are likely to remain intact.

We MSers call this "cog fog".

Though I've read that 50% of persons with MS can have some cognitive dysfunction, I question this number. It may be from MS, but sometimes we can be too quick to blame every problem we have on MS. Things like age, overload, fatigue, meds, and stress can affect these functions the same way. Nevertheless, it's real. My opinion: don't look for them, don't panic about them. There are things that can be done to manage them.

At my age, I can't live without post-its or notes, or remember the name of a movie I watched last week. My non-MS friends and I joke about these things all the time—we've joined the ranks of the golden years. Like anything with your body, if you don't use it, you'll lose it. Much is being reported about keeping your mind active by doing mental exercises such as crossword puzzles, jigsaw puzzles, or Sudoku as you grow older.

Other tips:

- Find things to challenge your brain. I learned a foreign language and really believe it helped keep my mind sharp.

- Focus on doing one task at a time in a distraction-free place.

- Too much noise, activity or confusion can be difficult to tolerate. I take "time-outs" by going into a quieter place, or I wear ear plugs.

- Ask family and friends to speak slower to give you more time to process information.

- Inquire about naltrexone. For some folks, low-dose naltrexone (LDN) may improve mental clarity and reduce brain fog since it acts on the nervous system. It's available, safe, and inexpensive because the dose is only 3 mg/day.

The Elephants in the Room
Part I: Mental and Behavioral Health

In recent years, mental and behavioral health have come to the forefront. Both are just as important as physical health. A deterioration of at least one of the three significantly impacts the other two. If left untreated, serious effects will result.

The good news is that it's finally getting the attention it deserves. Covid-19 has intensified the exposure of this trio. The bad news is that mental or behavioral health can be misunderstood, stressed too much, and greedy people capitalize on it.

Unfortunately, most folks do not understand the interplay between these three health areas. First, mental health and behavioral health are *not* the same. Mental health encompasses factors like your biology, psychological condition and habits. Behavioral health examines how your habits impact your overall physical and mental wellbeing.

For example, if the cause of depression is mental (e.g., neurological), then negative behaviors can follow. Treating the negative behaviors first may be the wrong path to go. Since MS affects the brain, antidepressants are commonly tried first. Learned misconceptions are also problematic. Sometimes if you tell people that you are depressed, they will automatically assume that having MS is getting you down. This may be true, but it may not be.

So, the right diagnosis and doctor (psychiatrist or psychologist) are critical. Going down the wrong path is dangerous, costly and time consuming. In my case, my neurologist (Dr. Excellent) addressed my depression and prescribed Prozac years ago.

Balance and moderation in quantity are necessary as well. Many times, I have shared that therapy beyond my physical needs has helped me through several dark times. I'll do just about anything to feel better and do better. I was lucky to have the right help, from the right place. for the right amount of time. Sadly, many people are bounced around for years without a solution to move forward.

In the past, if a person was seeing a psychiatrist or psychologist, it was hidden or not openly discussed. Getting mental help was generally a stigma and often a distorted problem. How many times have we heard the words "shrink" or "psycho"? Nowadays, I hear the news or see ads on TV about suicide and other difficulties that are not physical-health related. *Nevertheless, it still can be an elephant in the room.* If you tell someone you are seeing a psychiatrist or are in therapy, their expression tells it all.

In the same vein as physical health, homework is essential in finding the right help with the right people. Get *quality* help. The same rules apply as mentioned earlier (see *Doctors/Hospitals/Vaccines* chapter). Finding help in the top 10% of the arena, getting second opinions, if one doesn't work then find another…

What if the people we need to talk with won't communicate with us? Then find someone who will.

In the beginning of my MS in 1980, my family was in denial. I went straight to the local chapter of the National MS Society to get literature and meet others who had MS. Later, when both my husband and my mother couldn't talk to me about my MS, I went to a behavioral therapist who *understood MS* to help myself deal with these two important people in my life. Years later, I went to a psychologist again when deciding whether to give up my career. My MS was aggressive and progressing rapidly.

There's no question that people living with a person who is chronically ill, such as MS, is also living with it too. While open communication is essential for all involved, it unfortunately doesn't always happen effectively without having an "outside" person/s involved. Perceptions are different, emotions are involved, and more often than not, negative consequences result. Ideally, partner/family counseling is essential in most cases.

Realistically, there are obstacles with professional counseling.

1. Many people--whether they have the illness or not--do not want to go to counseling. As I explained, this was the case in my own personal situation. Though I pleaded with my family to go, it didn't happen. By going to counseling on my own, I learned much about interpersonal relationships plus how and where I could get support.

2. I believe it is imperative that a good, reputable therapist who *understands* MS is found. It's critical they understand the complications of MS and your specific new "normals". If they don't—which is often the case—you need to help teach them. Give them a copy of this book!

3. Many people unfortunately cannot afford therapy; however, many county health departments have resources available for financially strapped people and available online help is growing.

A sub-category of mental and behavioral health is abuse and addiction, which is *prevalent* in MS. Read on...

The Elephants in the Room
Part II: Abuse and Addiction

Physical Abuse

This subject is recognized often in movies, news, etc., mostly in the way of physical bruising, sexual assault, or even death. Often, the victim comes out of it as the hero in the movies; in reality, not so much.

This is tragic for sure, and for the victims it becomes a tangled mess of where to go and what to do. Especially when there are kids involved. There are places to run to like family/friends, the police, and safe houses. However, it is easier said than done. The victim lives in fear.

But a person's disability itself can provoke the abuser. Caregivers need to be chosen carefully.

A physically-abused person may not get out of the house enough for others to notice the visible signs. Symptoms are exacerbated, caused both the abuse and subsequently the MS. Advanced disability limits the avenues of how and where a person can go.

Lucky for me, I have never been subjected to this by anyone. I will leave the extensive information for another credible source. But if I was in this situation, I would follow my earliest instincts, gather my evidence, and then get out before it's too late.

Emotional Abuse

Emotional abuse is just as horrific as physical abuse. Victims live in chronic stress and fear. Again, symptoms are exacerbated by the abuse and subsequently the MS. It can kill too, in a different way. People with MS have a higher rate of abuse than average—perhaps as high as 50% of all relationships.

Most emotional abuse goes unnoticed and unreported. When the abuse takes place in private, there are no witnesses to validate your experience. Calling the police doesn't protect you like physical abuse would—there are no visible signs. Too often, family or friends can't/won't get involved. You and the entire family will "walk on eggshells" and adapt so as not to upset the abuser. Signs of depression, withdrawal, anxiety, etc. that result are blamed on the MS. It's a bad spot to be in, and becomes another elephant in the room.

Emotional abuse is when one person controls and dominates another. There becomes a power imbalance in abusive relationships where the abuser has all the power and the victim feels that they have none. Maybe it is screaming, swearing or downgrading you. Maybe it is neglecting or ignoring you. Maybe threats are made. Even if you are not getting smacked or punched, maybe they are being rough with you physically when they are assisting you. Maybe you are being teased, criticized, mocked relentlessly. *It hurts.*

> *See:* **Forms of Emotional and Verbal Abuse You May Be Overlooking** https://www.psychologytoday.com/us/blog/toxic-relationships/201704/forms-emotional-and-verbal-abuse-you-may-be-overlooking

Victims really *do* have the power in this situation to stop the emotional abuse, but it can be difficult. Once again, getting started is the hardest part. Trust me--you will be glad you did.

> **Dealing with Emotional Abuse**
> https://bit.ly/2TP2iaE

> **Emotionally Abusive Men and Women: Who Are They?**
> https://www.healthyplace.com/abuse/emotional-

psychological-abuse/emotionally-abusive-men-and-women-
who-are-they

- Find a good therapist through referral from a trusted source, like your doctor. You are not alone—reach out for help. Find the *right* therapist. In cases like these, seeing a therapist for solely depression/anxiety is the result, not the main root of the problem; meds alone will just mask it.

- Learn techniques to learn how to effectively set boundaries and diffuse the aggressive behaviors.

- Discreetly take notes, videos, or other things to support what is happening. Documenting things help assert that "it is not you".

I am an open book, and share experiences if it will help someone. It doesn't embarrass me. My husband's nature can be explosive; he will lose his temper easily or has little patience with things. So, he will yell and swear loudly, too often times directly at me. If I try to talk about it, he tells me I'm too sensitive and gets angrier. There would be more outbursts if I broke down. Truthfully, I admit that I *am* a sensitive person, especially when I'm tired and don't feel well. Crying is my release. I'd withdraw and drink too much. He refused counseling and I needed to do something.

One night after a horrible exchange, I drank too much. I ended up driving my power chair into a wall, knocked myself out, and ended up in the hospital with a bad concussion. It was a painful lesson.

I was recommended to a DBT group (dialectical behavior therapy). DBT goals are to teach people how to live in the moment, develop healthy ways to cope with stress, regulate their emotions, and improve their relationships with others.

Source: What Is Dialectical Behavior Therapy (DBT)? https://www.verywellmind.com/dialectical-behavior-therapy-1067402

My group was terrific; I was one of eight members, for a course of three months. Private insurance picked up the expense and I came away with whole toolkit of things. The group counselor also covered useful techniques like mindfulness, relaxation, and breathing.

Group membership was an amazing mix of people from the age of 17 to 70, varied levels of education and the reason for why they were there. Three girls were in college, three were employed, two suffered from depression, one was suicidal, one was raped, one had an eating disorder, two were bullied, one was bipolar.

Omg, I thought *I* had problems. Yet, we all needed help, bonded together and came out of it. The comraderies of sharing and empathizing with each other with a terrific counselor as a facilitator/educator was a new beginning.

Again, if you are the victim, or if you sense this problem exists with someone you care about, do something *now*. Remember, getting started is the hard part.

Scars from abuse are as deep as the damage from MS.

Note: I donated a copy of this book with this chapter bookmarked to my local police to educate them, so they can help victims of mental abuse if called. They needed the education/resources. Want to do the same for yours? Email me through my website www.DebbieMS.com and I'll send a book.

Addiction

A sub category of mental health is addiction; everyone knows what it is. There are all different types of addiction we hear about--drugs, opioids, alcohol, cigarettes, gambling, social media... Addiction to something is too often denied and obsessed about. Attention to this category has soared.

Too much of an addiction is unhealthy and will lead to bad consequences. We all know *that*, too. It's the addict that has to admit that their problem is real. I told my story of excessive drinking. Good thing I ran into a wall instead of another car.

Sometimes an addiction needs to be stopped; other times moderation or supervision is the key. Boundaries can be set. It's good sense. If under control, why deprive the person or make them feel guilty about it if logical steps are taken?

My 89-year-old mother still smokes 5-6 cigarettes a day and enjoys a nightcap. She wears an inflammable cape and my stepdad is there to supervise. When I was pregnant, my OB-GYN suggested I limit my cigarettes to five per day since I didn't think I could quit. He felt that the stress from quitting when not ready was just as risky as smoking ¼ pack a day. A solution that chased away guilt. I finally did quit a few years later. I haven't had a cigarette in 35 years, but I know if I just had one, I would start again.

I enjoy a scotch every night and have done it my whole life. It relaxes my body and calms my over-driven brain in the evening before bed. But I know that if the bottle were kept in my hands, there would be times when I would drink too excessively and perhaps run into another wall. So, the J & B sets on a high shelf, and a drink is served to me. It works. I take no drugs and have no other addictions, except reading.

Recognition. Moderation. Boundaries. Or quit, with support. It's good sense.

National Domestic Violence hotline 1-800-799-7233
https://www.domesticshelters.org /

The Elephants in the Room
Part III: Suicide

"I attempted it, but fortunately I survived."
(My personal diary, June 2008)

When I was a peer counselor for the MS Society, they always would give the folks with suicidal thoughts to me to talk with. I listened, I put myself in their shoes to understand why they were thinking about suicide, and I always managed to get them on a road to help themselves get out of that situation.

In recent years, this subject is emerging on the awareness front. There has been a rise in suicide by people in the armed services. And again, the Covid-19 pandemic was instrumental in bringing it to the forefront.

Yes, both awareness and attention have increased. However, too many times, the elephant stays in the closet until it is too late.

As mentioned previously, clinical depression is a serious issue to be dealt with and can be successfully treated. It is very common in MS, and if not treated, suicidal thoughts will begin to emerge. And it is nothing to be ashamed about. But suicidal thoughts are not always created by depression. MS is difficult to live with, and those that progress to the most advanced stages have their feelings about their dignity and quality of life to be understood. The ugliness of abuse drives people to the edge of the cliff, too.

I believe in euthanasia. My husband and I were caretakers for Grandma, who lived to be 102 years old in a nursing home. Her last ten years of life were spent in bed—she was blind and she couldn't walk. She emigrated from the Slovakia in 1916 and spoke limited, broken English. Her mind was sharp as a pin, but her pain almost unbearable. Her husband, daughter, son, friends had all died; she prayed "Jesus, take me" every day. Every week we visited her; we also visited many other people around her in the same situation. I know what quality of life is and what it is not. Why shouldn't people be allowed to decide for themselves what to do with their own life without being scorned?

I had suicidal thoughts a few times over the years, but it was always the thought of my son that prevented me from going through with it. I felt great love and a responsibility to raise him to at least eighteen years of age. If I brought the subject of suicide up to someone in my family to talk about, I was cut off at the pass immediately. It was unthinkable that I would do something like that.

Thirteen years ago, I snapped. I wasn't depressed, and it wasn't premeditated. I was tired of being sick, and sick of being tired. My husband and I had an argument, as all married couples do, but I was feeling awful and vulnerable. I took the dog around the block for a walk and I thought: "I have no more obligations, I have been successful in life, and I'm not going to take any of this crap anymore." I went home. As I lay in bed, I took an overdose of pills. I knew from the internet what to do. And I wanted to do it while I still could. I didn't want to end up in Grandma's position.

My son had come into my bedroom when I was on the verge of unconsciousness and called 911. I ended up being in the psyche ward only three days. The head of the department kept insisting I was suffering from depression and was pushing me to say and do things I didn't want to do. I kept insisting I wasn't depressed, that my buttons were pushed and I just snapped. I got up daily, did my exercises, put on my makeup and cheerfully attended all my group and therapy appointments. They gave me an early release, but I think it was really because none of the bathrooms in the rooms were handicapped accessible, and the main accessible bathroom they had at the front desk was being used as a storage facility! I had made a fuss about it and could have caused a lot of trouble. They let me go, so I let *it* go.

Anyway, when I talked to my immediate family, it was uncomfortable. They didn't know what to say to me and just small talked. My distraught husband said to please never do this again. None of my neighbors approached me for quite some time when I got home, despite the fact they were all around when the ambulance and fire trucks had come to the house.

It was my son who would talk about it, usually after a few drinks, and I realized what a disturbing, profound effect it had on him. He told me I did major damage to him emotionally, and to this day, the effects are still there. I made a terrible, selfish mistake and because of him, I will not think about it again. I've moved on in life, continuing to enjoy things and find other things to accomplish, like writing this book.

People really don't know what to say, or ask, or react about suicide. My family never brought up the subject of suicide since, so I didn't bother telling anyone else because I knew the reaction I would get. I didn't want to make anyone feel uncomfortable. But I misjudged.

When I was catching up on the phone one day with one of my best friends, Rita, I told her about my overdose. She "got" it when we talked about it and asked me if I was going to put it in my book. When I replied no, she challenged me and said "why not?". She's right.

I do get it, and *it needs to be an open subject for everyone--the person with MS, their friends, family, and doctors. And a person with MS needs to think through thoroughly and talk about it, because it is a final decision.*

Most people don't get a second chance like I did.

Note: Call the U.S. National Suicide Prevention Lifeline at 800-273-TALK (8255), a free, 24/7 service that can provide suicidal persons or those around them with support, information and resources. (Source: National Institute of Mental Health.)

Employment/Long-Term Disability

There is a silver lining in every cloud.

To tell or not to tell?

When newly diagnosed, people often wonder if they should tell their employer about their diagnosis. There are pros and cons to each side. Despite what folks tell you about your rights and protection under the law, we all know there are ways to get around discrimination. Sadly, tactics such as overloading your workload, undermining your performance, or eliminating your position are used.

My opinion? I believe it comes down to trust and safety. Who can you trust with what information, and how safe are you in your working environment?

When I was diagnosed, I was working as a manager in a major bank. Fortunately, I strongly felt I could confidentially talk to my immediate manager and a couple of fellow associates. I had fatigue and bathroom issues, but for the most part I looked like a normal person. There was that uncertainty though, about what might happen to me going forward.

Then, I notified the nursing department, and arranged to rest in one of their beds during my lunch hour. Finally, I notified the security department in case the building had to be evacuated for some reason; working on the 13th floor, there was no way I would be able to exit via the stairways.

Yep, it happened. A fire started in the copy room on the floor and everyone was told to evacuate. While I waiting for the firemen with the stretcher to rescue me, the fire was contained and I didn't have to be carried to ground level. Ha—the irony of that floor number! It was unlucky, but I ended up lucky.

Employment

The Covid-19 pandemic was tough on jobs for sure. A positive outcome though was the amazing transformation in the workplace. Technology, zoom meetings and working-at-home are in a place that wasn't there prior to it. The transition was cumbersome, but the dynamics in the work and marketplace created many possibilities to do things without having to leave the house.

Job interviews and applications for employment help folks with physical difficulties. Emerging new opportunities like telehealth appointments and home deliveries save time and energy. The list goes on…

But what if you have to continue working in an office or place outside the home, and your MS has caused advanced physical and mental difficulties? Maybe your financial or benefits situation requires you to continue working.

What to know about asking for work accommodations?

- Your right to accommodations depends on your specific employer and disability status.

- In the U.S., many employers are legally required to provide reasonable accommodations for disabled employees. More information about your rights can be found through the U.S. Department of Labor's Job Accommodation Network https://askjan.org/publications/individuals/employee-guide.cfm

Some reasonable accommodations for comfort and safety may include:

- transfer from full-time to part-time work
- work from home, full-time or part-time
- adjustment of work responsibilities
- extra time off for sick leave or medical appointments

- moving your parking place for better accessibility

Long-Term Disability Insurance

I started this section many times, and decided to start this subject with my own story as to how I made the decision, what I went through, and how I coped. It was a difficult, painful decision and adjustment. I needed tons of support. Ultimately, I made the decision alone, and in the end, it worked out for me.

Seven years after my first MS occurrence, I was working full time in a demanding, responsible position for a large bank. My son was four years old, and the stressful, physical daily demands of the job, motherhood, and running a household were causing my symptoms to worsen. Daily, I would eat a packed sandwich at my desk and then go to the nurses' station to lie down for an hour. My job performance and home life were suffering.

One day, after wetting the bed during a nap at the nurses' station, I could barely walk back to my desk even though I was using a cane. Breaking down, I called my neurologist and explained what was happening. He said he would make arrangements to admit me into the hospital immediately for treatment. I told my manager why I was leaving, turned and walked out. It happened that fast.

My doctor admitted me for a two-week rest, with daily injections of ACTH. This is a steroid that was used at that time, followed by prednisone to help reduce the severity and duration of a flare-up. (Note: ACTH treatment, now known as Acthar Gel, has re-emerged again recently.) At the point when I had called my neurologist, I was wetting the bed every night, losing control of my bowels intermittently, and experiencing severe eye pain from optic neuritis. It had been three years already since I began wetting the bed. I was dragging my left leg, and the weakness and spasticity in my legs had limited my walking ability to two blocks. And there was much more.

After two weeks, I was feeling emotionally better but many physical problems remained; so, I went on short-term disability. I found an excellent urologist whose team taught me how to do self-Catherization, bladder and bowel management. Hospital testing showed I now had a neurogenic bladder. I needed physical therapy for walking. It was impossible to walk without using a cane or holding onto a wall or furniture. Fatigue was overwhelming when I would do anything physical over an hour.

Three months later, I was proficient at the bladder/bowel management, but the gait problems showed little improvement. I learned how to manage my spasticity through stretching, exercise and medication, but my walking was limited due to my loss of balance, coordination and weakness. The fatigue remained.

My company was pushing me for a decision about my return date. If I was not going to return, then I would have to apply for disability. I was fortunate I had a good relationship with my manager, who had confided in me that I should really think about leaving and going on long-term disability. If I went back to work, I faced the possibility that my job could be eliminated. We were good friends, and we both knew that companies will find ways to eliminate you no matter what the ADA (Americans with Disability Act) laws say. I was working in a corporate world—still largely a "man's" world in the banking industry—and I knew after years of being in key management positions how they did unethical things and got around it.

I was the primary breadwinner, earning very good money. How could we make it financially on so much less money if I went on disability? I would be giving up my career—nobody would hire me if I decided to try to get back into the workforce. How could I give up everything I worked so hard for? Again, I didn't care what the ADA laws said about hiring people with disabilities and making necessary accommodations for their special needs—the reality is that there is always somebody "more qualified". What could I do, going forward? I was only 32 years old.

I scheduled an appointment with my neurologist (Dr. Excellent) to discuss this. He minced no words in saying that it was the chronic stress and fatigue that brought me down so fast and severely. I had much residual damage and I shouldn't expect much function to return. There was no crystal ball to tell me when the next flare-up would be and how long it would last. We already knew how much neurological damage I suffered in just seven years. I had to think about my health, my priorities. I had a child to raise.

Furthermore, if I went on disability, it would have to be a permanent decision. Getting approved for disability was extremely difficult at that time for a person with MS. Things like ataxia and fatigue were not considered disabling.

I was faced with a stressful situation whichever choice I made. In the end I had to put myself and my health first. Something needed to be done to slow down the rapid progression of the disease—to try and stabilize and prevent further damage until a cure could be found. I was so frightened to think if I was this bad after seven years, what would happen and where would I be in the next seven years?

Fortunately, I was approved for social security the first time I applied. I cut house-cleaning services and didn't have caretaker expenses anymore since I could be at home with my son full-time. My husband was working and had a good healthcare benefit plan which was a relief. And when you have to cut the budget to make ends meet, it's amazing what you can learn to live without.

While I had reduced stress by being able to stay home and rest more, different stresses took over. The first had to do with receiving a government entitlement. The second had to do with my self-esteem. Although I was happy to be able to be a stay-at-home mom, I had worked all my life and felt I should be doing something more, especially when my son started kindergarten.

Counseling helped to address both of these issues. I had many talents that I could put to good use by volunteering when I felt up to it. I contacted the National MS Society to discuss opportunities there, and I got involved at my son's school. This sounds crazy, but it felt good to be able to "give back" as a way to "earn" my benefits. As time went on, I continued to have problems with MS symptoms and flare-ups, but it reassured me that I deserved and needed to be on disability. Being home gave me the opportunity to learn how to take care of myself. It was the right decision.

Unfortunately, at the present time, I know that getting LTD can still be difficult.

When I'm asked, "What should I do if I'm thinking about applying for long-term disability benefits?" these are my suggestions:

- Document *everything*—symptoms, flare-ups, medications/treatments taken, all doctors/other professional help visits, etc.—and *be specific* (when, what, frequency, duration, why, results/non-results, side effects…).

- Schedule at least two visits to your neurologist/year. Consider seeing a professional therapist for depression and other emotional problems you may be experiencing; consult with them about prescriptions for an antidepressant, anxiety, or sleep.

- Make sure you have a good, supportive neurologist—my neurologist knew exactly what to write and explain specifically on required paperwork to get me approved.

- When completing disability documents, include the following points.

  - In addition to the gait, vision, bladder/bowel, sleep, fatigue and emotional problems, you need to be specific with pain, coordination, weakness and balance problems.
  - Show that you are unable to stand or sit more than an hour or two at a time; and it's necessary to lie down at least every two hours.
  - Explain that not only are you unable to do *your* current job, but *any* job. (Like selling movie tickets!)
  - Detail how quickly you become incapacitated and how nauseated and sleepy you get from medication/treatments you are on.

- Once you get on disability benefits, *stay* on them. The unpredictability of a MS flare-up and the extent and duration of its impact can happen overnight.

Note: To obtain information about Social Security Disability, you can call your local social security office, or go online at www.socialsecurity.gov.

Video - Social Security Disability Law Updates for the MS Community
https://bit.ly/378RjMI MS News and Views

Vitamins/Supplements/Diet

You are what you eat—er, sometimes.

Let me begin by saying vitamins and supplements are not a replacement for healthy foods. But there are good reasons to take certain vitamins for an MSer, especially as you get older.

So, which ones to take and why?

- **Vitamin D**--Research has shown that people with MS have lower levels, increasing our risk for MS. Nowadays, neurologists will recommend taking 1000-2000 IU daily. Vitamin D is also needed to absorb calcium, needed for strong bones. Our ability to turn sunlight into vitamin D declines as we age. Aging also hinders Vitamin D absorption in its natural forms. *

- **Calcium**—This is needed for strong bones and teeth. Maintaining recommended calcium levels are particularly important for MSers who take steroids, have reduced their dairy intake, and to help prevent osteoporosis in aging. As a small-framed woman, I have always taken 1000-2000 mg. daily.

- **B12**—Having an essential role in nerve function/immune health, lacking this vitamin is associated with things like depression, decreased cognition and digestive issues. As we get older, our ability to absorb B12 slows. It's also worthwhile to know that you can't get B12 from plants. So, beware if you are vegan.

https://content.govdelivery.com/accounts/USNIHODS/bulletins/2e87b01

- **Vitamin C**—Low levels are rare in the average person. As mentioned previously, however, a daily intake of 500-1000 mg. daily is helpful in preventing urinary tract infections for folks with neurogenic bladders.

- **Probiotics**—A daily intake is helpful in keeping your gut healthy and balanced, a common problem for MSers. (See *Plumbing III: The Gut* chapter.)

*Caution—only take recommended amounts of D and B12; excess amounts can be harmful since the body can only absorb so much and can't eliminate the excess of these. No worries with vitamin C; your body will get rid of any excess.

Tip: Check out Life Extension strontium caps for bone health and density. I have taken strontium daily (750 mg.) for five years (for osteoporosis), and my bone-density exams have shown an increase in bone density! Info/references: https://articflex.com/strontium-vs-calcium/

Diet

Research has clarified the influence of inflammation on neurologic conditions like MS. An anti-inflammatory diet likely enhances brain health. This includes physical and mental health, in more ways than just the neurological system. (i.e., What's good for your brain, is good for your health.) So, it makes sense to have an anti-inflammatory diet *and* lifestyle.

Earlier, I suggested trying a Mediterranean diet. Google away to learn more about this diet, and other specific diet information. To enhance brain health, see my blog post *Brain Health: What to Know, What to Do?* in the Debbie's Favorite Blog Posts section in the back of this book.

My last words on diets.

Many persons with MS are advocates for different diets to follow, what you "should" eat/not eat, or what supplements to take. Some people find that dairy products are troublesome. Bottom line? If certain foods help you feel better, listen to your body and use your intelligence. Do minimal changes at a time. Keep a journal. Moderation and balance are key.

In the meantime, the good news is that more research is being done for the effects of diet on MS.

PART IV

WHAT ELSE IS HELPFUL TO KNOW?

Making Decisions when Managing MS

"I remained firm with the neurologist by confidently telling him, "No, I'm not going through that again." (Jessie Ace, DISabled to Enabled, Multiple Sclerosis Today, June 1, 2021)

Throughout this book, I have commented on this subject, but I thought a catch-all chapter may be a worthy reference. As the saying goes, "Sometimes you can lose sight of the forest through the trees."

In many online MS discussion groups, participants discuss what is the best thing to do or take for MS, and what is bunk. Subjects range from treatments, vaccines, diet, and stress to exercise, experimental drugs and alternative medicine.

While these groups and other resources such as newsletters and articles from accredited sources are valuable, relying on a single source or opinion is dangerous. So, it makes sense to collect information on a subject from as many sources as possible.

If someone seeks information from MS organizations or medical websites, a standard directive is "Ask your doctor." Of course, your doctor's opinion is valuable. But keep these thoughts in mind:

- Are you confident with just one opinion? For example, when I was deciding what to about the Shingrix vaccine, I initially researched the vaccine from diverse, credible online sources. Then I asked both my neurologist and PCP about it. Finally, I asked other MSers and "normal" people I knew who received the vaccine about their experiences.

- How confident are you with your doctor(s) opinion? Rate your confidence on a scale of one to ten. If the answer is a five, get another opinion.

- If you ask your doctor about treatments, most will recommend something for symptoms, for relapses, and long-term disease modifying therapies as long as there are no contraindications. There are two reasons for this:
  - They want to help you feel better and try to prevent you from getting worse. In addition, doctors certainly don't have the time to educate you or answer a lot of questions, especially if it is out of their area of expertise. They will refer you instead to physical/occupational therapy, other specialists, pain clinics, etc.
  - Relative to prescribing drugs (and vaccines), doctors rely on scientific evidence. They will send you off with referrals, scripts, tests, etc.

- If you ask something about body wellness for MS, they will generally agree that things such as exercise and proper diet are good for you. They will not address *specific* topics because there is not sufficient scientific evidence to determine the positive/negative impact on MS. For example, don't expect a specific answer to "Is Wahl's the best type of diet to follow?"

So, when you need to make a decision regarding something about your MS and are stuck, what should you do?

Personally, I practice logic and balance for both my body's wellness and medications I choose to use. I ask myself these questions:

- Does it make me feel better?
- What are the short/long term risks of doing or not doing something?
- Do the benefits outweigh the risks that I am willing to take?
- Do the overall pros outweigh the cons?

- Am I doing everything I can possibly do to keep my immune health strong?
- Did I gather enough research from reliable sources to help me make *my* decision?

If my instincts cause me to feel unsure, then I follow my mantra, *"When in doubt, don't!"* It's helpful to take a pause and think through it again another time.

When starting something new, keep journals of what you do, what's going on, and how you feel. This habit will be a good reference tool for both yourself and upcoming office visits.

Once again, there are no absolute rights or wrongs. I listen to my body and know it well, but I leave myself open to try something new if I feel it is safe and I have nothing to lose by trying. Like everyone else with MS, I want to feel better and get better.

Final decisions are made by me. I am the one who has to live with my body.

How to Deal with People

There are more good people than schmucks in the world.
There's a way to handle both. I've learned to lie, pretend
and be a good actress. I like people, and I need people.

- **Being honest and dishonest.**

  When someone asks me how I'm doing, I vary my responses depending on who I'm talking to. If it's a stranger or an acquaintance, I always say, "Fine, and how are you?" even if I am in the foulest mood. Why ruin their day, or in today's world, get somebody really irritated? I wouldn't risk being a smart-butt to someone, and besides, I would just make it worse for others who are in a wheelchair or disabled.

  If it's a good friend and if I'm down, I'll lie and say "I'm fine," or "I'm hanging in there…" Other times, I let my hair down. My friends truly want to know how I'm doing, but I don't want to complain every time I talk to them. Who likes that?

  That also goes for my close family who don't live with me. At home, I let my husband know if I'm doing well or not. If I'm having a bad day, it's hard for him to take it, so I usually keep my distance and do my own thing. When my son was growing up, I hid my feelings a lot because I didn't want him to worry about mom being sick. But I learned later it was also important to say "Mom's really tired today" once in a while.

- **Smiles and kindness go a long way.**

    Even if you feel crabby, fake a smile anyway. We need people and most of us like to interact with people. I'm almost always nice and smiling at people. When I ask for help, which in my case I have to ask for help a lot, I get what I need with a smile back. If I'm in a grocery store and can't reach an item, I'll nicely ask "When you have a moment, would you reach something for me?" I always get help, usually followed by the offer to let them know if I need anything else.

    When I was in the hospital last year, even though I felt miserable I always was kind and patient with the nurses. The nurses would actually give me extra attention, because they would remark how cranky everyone else was. They would sometimes hang out for a few minutes to yak, which actually elevated my moods. It's hard to do when you yourself are feeling so miserable, but the positive responses back are worth it.

- **You set the tone and put people at ease.**

    Many people feel uncomfortable around a disabled person, or don't know what to say. If I'm comfortable, it automatically makes them feel comfortable. This is easy for me, because, I've lived with MS for so long and been in a wheelchair/scooter for so many years; I actually forget that I'm in one and don't think about it. So, I always start with a smile, maybe nod, wave, or say a cheery expression about the weather depending on where I am or what I'm doing. I recently was in a grocery line and the basket attached to the front of my scooter was filled. The woman in front of me turned around as I was unloading, and I looked up at her, smiled and said 'hi'. She very timidly asked if she could help me unload. I thanked her and remarked that I'd love the help. She proceeded to say that she's afraid to ask people in my position because many become indignant and want to do it themselves. I told her to go ahead and keep on asking; just blow off the others because she either got them at a bad moment or they just had the wrong attitude.

- **Let people help.**

  They want to and many of them don't know how. Even if I don't actually need the help when people offer, I let them help anyway. It makes them feel good. Many times, people want to help but it's up to us to tell them how to help. There are many things I am able to do on my own—like getting dressed or washing clothes. But if someone can put my shoes on for me or empty the clothes out of the washer, then why not? It's less fatiguing for me, and it makes the person feel better because they don't have to watch me struggle to do something.

- **Show your manners and your gratefulness.**

  Just like smiles, "please" and "thank you" go a long way. Sadly, in today's society, many people don't have manners but I have learned to rise above that and it is amazing how I will get a positive response. If I want or need something, I always start off by saying, "When you have time, will you please…?" instead of demanding and insisting for things right away. (Of course, it's different if you've just fallen down on the floor!)

  Similarly, everyone likes to feel appreciated, and just sincerely saying thank you is not only the right thing to do, but when you need to ask for something again from someone, you'll get it without grumbling. I usually go much further however. I always acknowledge people who help me regularly with more than just a verbal thanks. I send cards, notes of gratitude, give gifts at Christmastime to even doctors' offices, receptionists… It doesn't have to be expensive. There are many people who help me in many ways, and I am so very grateful. It's my nature to do this, but the payback is always tenfold.

  When I call my doctor's office, guess who gets immediate attention? The other side of it is that sometimes I am in such a bad mood and feel so awful, that I lash out at people. Later, if it's someone I care about, I apologize. If it was a stranger that I jumped all over, oh well, I'll never see them again (so now *I'm* the schmuck) and hopefully not get shot in the meantime.

- **What about those people who park in handicapped parking places illegally, or use the handicapped toilet stalls when they are normal?**

  I used to get all in a huff about it, but learned over time, it is not worth getting all stressed out over. These people are inconsiderate schmucks, and they won't change or care if you scream at them. Instead, write their plate number down and turn them in if you want to take action, or find the nearest security officer and point them out. (Phoenix has a phone number that can be called to report offenders: 602-534-space; check with your city about this.)

  Now, if I'm in a crowded bathroom with a line and a normal person is using a handicapped stall, I don't get all ruffled, because generally when the person comes out, the waiting line urges me forward. But, if I'm in an empty restroom and the only stall being used is the handicapped one by a normal person, it does tick me off and my look is enough to make the guilty person slink out of the room quickly. What else can you do with these jerks?

- **The way you approach somebody about a problem often will result in how (or if) that problem will be resolved.**

  I know this is another commonsense thing, but it is true. If you act like a jerk, you will probably not get what you want. Earlier this year I booked a handicapped room at a hotel, and asked my usual one hundred questions about the room before I booked. One of the things I specifically asked about was the height of the bed. I know high beds are fashionable these days, but for someone in a wheelchair, this is a problem. I was assured that the bed was a normal height.

  When I checked into my room, you guessed it. The bed was very high, and since I was travelling alone, there was no way I was going to be able to get in and out of it. I called the front desk and asked for a manager to please come to my room. I nicely demonstrated my dilemma, and asked them to take out the six or eight-inch frame and lower the bed. They did it, and made some other arrangements to the room that I needed. I graciously thanked the manager and she graciously thanked me for being so nice about it, adding that many people are so rude and quick to complain.

Sure, I could have accused them about ADA standards but what good would it do? I got what I wanted, plus three days of exceptional service that followed for anything I needed. Realistically, if I complained to an agency, nothing would have ever have been done about it.

- **Be an educator.**

Fortunately, most people nowadays are aware of MS, but still don't really understand it or know what it is. That includes even doctors, or other people in the health field.

Once when I had to get a mole removed from my lower leg, I had to explain to the dermatologist about the spasticity in my lower leg. Her assistant and I were going to have to hold onto the leg very tightly while she administered the shot to numb my leg, or else it would jerk quickly and rapidly. If I'm having an X-ray done, I talk to the tech beforehand to discuss the best way for me to move my body around. The nursing staff in the infirmary at the amusement park where I went to take a nap and get ice packs had no idea that heat could cause such havoc in a MSer.

It is important to help kids understand it. When I tutored at schools and churches, I showed the kids how my hand controls worked, let them bring a manual wheelchair to my car, help carry my things for me, and open the doors for me.

When I explain what MS is, I use the word "disorder" rather than "disease". The word "disease" connotes that it's contagious, and I'm careful to explain that you can't "catch" MS or die from it; most people don't end up in wheelchairs or have pain from it. (They don't have to know *that* or specific details.) Even though there is no cure for MS, there are many things a person can take or do to help with the symptoms. *The simpler the explanation, the better it is.*

When I was younger, adults approached me from time to time when I was out and about on my scooter and asked what kind of accident I had, or why I used a scooter since "I looked so good". I have no problem taking the time to explain I have MS, and often people will remark that they know someone who has it but really don't understand it. When I say I've had it for 31 years, they are flabbergasted and begin asking me many questions about MS.

- **There will be people who can't accept that you have MS.**

    Sadly, there will be spouses and family members who can't accept it, and divorce rates are high. I have family members who have never read anything about MS, but will mention something only if there's some new study or drug being tested. It hurts. You can't make them accept it or read something if they don't want to.

    If it seriously bothers you emotionally, professional counseling does help. I can personally vouch for that. I learned to find support and acceptance by talking to other MSers, friends, and people I met volunteering with the MS Society.

- **Try not to look too good or be too independent.**

    It could backfire on you. I always took great care to look good, be as independent as possible and not complain. But then when a particularly bad day or flare-up occurred, I would hear "What's *wrong* with her?" My family around me were at a loss as to what to do, and was annoyed with me. Or, there was always an expectation that I would "find a way" or "work it out"; and somehow, I would bounce back and take care of things again.

    If I had a few days of downtime, the dishes would continue to pile up in the sink, the mail would continually get stacked and unopened, and the laundry basket would flow over. Not anymore! I'm much better at looking like a slob, taking daily naps and asking someone to go for Chinese take-out. Old habits are slow and hard to change, but it can be done.

- **If there is something you want or need from someone, attitude is everything.**

  And don't burn bridges—you never know when you will need that person someday.

Now let's consider the other viewpoint—how someone can deal with the person with MS...

How to Deal with a Person with MS

"It's not easy to deal with a person with MS.
They can be mean, cranky, and difficult to handle.
Do you have any suggestions?"
(*A question by a nurse with hospital staff at a NMSS*
information session on MS, October, 1992)

Very true, and quite often, it's *not* easy to deal with a person with MS. We *are* mean and cranky because we don't feel well, we are tired, and we are scared. Yeah, the person with MS is living with the disease, but so are the people who live with and interact with that person.

What to do?

- **Be compassionate and empathetic, *not* sympathetic or rough in your actions and language.**

    Don't feel sorry for a person with MS, but *learn to understand what MS is all about* and that will help you figure out what to do and how to (re)act. It's not good to constantly remark how sorry you feel for so-and-so or wait on a person with MS constantly. But telling someone, for example, to "quit complaining, get a grip, and learn to live with it" will generate additional stress and negativity. Being offensive will result in less cooperation. Often, a simple hug works wonders. Visualize putting yourselves in their shoes.

- **Ask if you can help and how you can help.**

  Do they need a babysitter, help with dinner or laundry, just some company, or something from the store? If you offer, make sure you follow through with it. If you see them struggling to do something, like putting on a sock, ask if you can help them. If they say "no", let it go. Don't take it personally.

- **Ask if they would like to talk—about what hurts, what's bothering them, about anything.**

  If they say yes, then *listen*. If they say 'no', ask them if they would like to talk to someone else, such as a peer counselor. If they say 'no', let it go. Again, don't take it personally. More often than not, they need someone to listen to them.

- **Don't be pushy with advice, but ask if they *want* advice.**

  If the answer is 'yes', make it a two-way conversation. *But—*

  - If you have noticed signs of depression or new symptoms that have gone on for more than several days, then suggest they talk to their neurologist about it. Offer to make the appointment and go with them.
  - Refer to the "Bad days vs. Flare-ups" chapter and review the checklist. If you have observed something that could be causing problems, make a suggestion about it (e.g., Are you having trouble sleeping? Are you feeling hot? Are you on a new medication?)

- **Let them vent if they have to.**

  If they start yelling or crying, ask if they want you to stay, leave, or give them a hug.

- **Inspiration vs. Reality.**

  Inspiration is vital. However, there are times when MSers are so sick or fatigued, they don't want cheerleading, humor, or advice.

- **Don't make comparisons to others or suggest that things could be a lot worse.**

    From my experience, these types of comments create more negative reactions than positive ones.

- **Do you know someone newly diagnosed who is in denial, won't see a doctor, or talk about it?**

    Just quietly hand them this book and walk away.

- **If you live with the person with MS, make sure *you* get your space, get out, or take a time-out.**

    You are living with MS too, like it or not. There are support groups for caregivers and others living with MSers; or in general, chronic illnesses. Contact the local chapter of the National MS Society, other MS associations, or search the internet for support groups in your area. *You need peers too—those who are in your shoes.* A goal is to minimize stress and anxiety as much as possible for everyone involved. Communicate and work out things together, because you *are* in this together.

In summary, encourage them to do anything to help make them feel better physically, mentally or emotionally. It could be as simple as taking a shower, lowering the thermostat, or telling them how much you care. And, if they *do* look good, say it this way: "I know you feel like crap, but you *do* look good!

This list is for family, friends, co-workers, health care professionals...i.e., the people we associate with in our lives. While it seems to be simple and logical, it is amazing how many folks say the wrong things or don't even know what to say.

(See *MS and Your Relationships* in Debbie's Favorite Blog Posts section at the end of this book.)

Positives to Having MS

Attitude is everything. Like I said before, I am an optimistic person and often think there is something good that can come out of a negative thing. There are advantages to having MS.

- **You become more careful about your health.**

    I have learned to take care of myself--I can't afford to get sick because of the negative effect illness can have on MS. My internist said to me once during a routine check-up "Don't take this wrong, Deb, but you are the healthiest patient I've seen all day!"

    Many normal people in their younger years are so busy with their jobs, their families, and their households they make themselves the last priority on the list. I like to use the example of the video overview airlines give prior to takeoff. When oxygen masks drop, parents should always put theirs on first, and then take care of their kids. You work better and faster, and don't risk passing out while trying to take care of your kids. It's common sense.

    I'm the glue in my household, and if I don't put myself as top priority health wise, everything would be much worse, including me.

- **You are more in tune with your body.**

    A person with MS is more likely to notice things out of the ordinary, take preventative measures and check for things a normal person would likely ignore or not think about. I was in my early 30's when I decided to see a specialist about a dark mole on my back. It turned out to be a malignant melanoma, and I had to have it removed within the week. Otherwise, as my dermatologist put it, I would be dead in six months.

Paying attention to your body also enables you to take action faster if a cold, infection or virus starts brewing. I know immediately when I have a UTI or sinus infection, so that I get antibiotics within that day before it escalates and becomes a major problem. Infections lead to flare-ups and complications.

- **You take nothing for granted.**

My health is #1, and if I'm feeling good on a particular day, I notice it and am glad for it. Things could always be/get worse and that makes me appreciate what I am able to do or have. Yeah, it's a bummer that I don't walk anymore, but I'm glad for new treatments, scooters, power chairs, accessibility and everything that is available that wasn't even as recently as 30 or 40 years ago.

- **Living with MS has taught me that it's okay to makes mistakes and not to be perfect; to focus on what really is important.**

Everyone makes mistakes and we learn from them. In my teens and early twenties, I was always trying to be perfect or dwelled on insignificant things. Not earning an "A" or cleaning my windows caused unnecessary stress. Years later, when my son sneezed while eating pureed beets in his high chair, my husband freaked since he was the one who was feeding him. I busted out laughing—what else was there to do? It's only beets. (Maybe part of it was motherhood?) When writing this book, I focused on what to say and how to say it. Sure, I want it completed as best as possible, but I'm not going to lose sleep if I find some editing errors after it's published. (Maybe part of it is being a senior?) I'm glad I don't sweat the small stuff, but focus instead on what *really* matters. Well, usually.

- **Living for the day.**

  In early adulthood, I never stopped to "smell the roses." I was always on the go doing what needed to be done. Now, I will postpone mundane home chores to enjoy a lunch with girlfriends, sit on the patio and watch the birds, or gab with the neighbors. Some people can do this anyway, and I always wished I had that laid-back attitude. But now, if I wake up and feel good, I take advantage of it—even if it's something that will lead to a "pay day" tomorrow. Last year when I was tutoring a group of kids at the church, a rare rainstorm came. Since we get so few days of rain in Phoenix, I told the kids to go out and play in the rain. They were ecstatic. We could always have class, but we can't always play in the rain. We all stopped and smelled the roses that day! We made up the work another time.

- **Planning for the future.**

  The unpredictability of the nature and course of MS always leaves us to wonder, "Where will I will be in one year? five years? ten years?" I was always a planner and organizer by nature, and being in tune with my body enabled me to have the foresight to do things while I had the opportunity.

  When my balance and gait got so poor, I arranged a trip to the shore one September when the weather was cooler so that I could have my last walk on the beach. When I knew I was near the time when I could no longer swim in the ocean, I arranged a trip to the ocean and had the lifeguards carry me into the water to jump waves for the last time. While this may sound sad, I wanted to get my last chances in and then I could move onto other things. There are always other things.

  My husband and I bought an accessible RV 17 years ago, and we have enjoyed so many places and National Parks. (See *tip* below.) It's a comfortable way for me to travel—always having the bathroom and bed available. We worked hard so that he could retire early, and we are doing our retirement stuff now. We took a rail trip through Alaska and a plane ride over the Grand Canyon.

We are nature, history and museum lovers, and will do what we can now, while we can.

Tip: There is something called an *Access Pass* for citizens or permanent residents of the United States who have been medically determined to have a permanent disability. It provides free access to, and use of, any Federal recreation site that charges an Entrance or Standard Amenity Fee and provides a discount on some Expanded Amenity Fees. For more information, the website is www.us-parks.com/golden-access-passport.html.

- **You (can) develop mental toughness.**

  Sometimes people have asked me, "How do you do it?" Harvey MacKay says it best: * *Mental toughness grows in the moments when you think you can't go on, but you keep going anyway. Anyone can give up. But to hold it together when everyone else would understand if you fell apart—that's true mental toughness.*

  How? You focus only on what you can control. You learn from your failures, but don't dwell on them. You ask for advice and feedback. That's how a person survives; they have grit and resilience. **

  I have found it impressive that so many MSers learn to develop this.

*Harvey Mackay is the author of the New York Times best-seller "Swim With the Sharks Without Being Eaten Alive." He can be reached through his website, harveymackay.com

**15 Habits of Mentally Tough People
  https://www.entrepreneur.com/article/248234

Personal Choices

Throughout the journey in everyone's life, difficult choices have to be made.

These were choices I made solely due to my MS, and fortunately for me, they were correct choices.

- **I chose to move to the desert.**

   I was living in Pittsburgh, a very humid, hilly, inaccessible city, with winters that were long and tough. My house had three floors, built on a hillside, without a bathroom on the main floor. I had two stair glides, used an electric wheelchair on the main floor, a walker upstairs and a scooter in my basement area to get to the washer and garage. I was constantly transferring and starting to fall quite often. I needed to make a move, and decided I would do it when my son graduated from high school, but the big question was "Where?"

   I had lived in Pittsburgh my entire life, and some of my family, all my friends and health care professionals were there. My husband had almost four more years to go before he could retire. After a lot of thought and research, the bold decision to move to Glendale, Arizona was made. At that time, I was forty-five years old and my son had just started his senior year in high school. I have an aunt and uncle who live in Phoenix, so I booked a trip there and they were tremendous in helping us check it out and make it happen.

The climate is dry with low humidity which makes me feel so much better. My house has a built-in pool that I use eight months out of the year for therapy, and there is accessibility all around me. I have a one floor home, live on an accessible bus line, and use disability door-to-door transportation service offered by the city. Within a quarter mile from my home are two shopping centers, a hospital and many medical facilities that I can drive my scooter to. No hills, no winters. During the summer when it is extremely hot, I do my swimming and other outdoor activities at the crack of dawn and stay indoors in air conditioning the rest of the time. I found utopia.

My son decided to go to Arizona State University. My husband and I decided that he would stay in Pittsburgh until he retired, which was extremely important to both of us, and that I would live alone in Glendale. I was confident I could manage. Between his vacation time and family leave, he was able to come to Glendale several times each year. We succeeded. It has been the right move for me from a health standpoint--both physically and emotionally. And I love Arizona as much as Pittsburgh.

- **I chose not to walk anymore.**

  When I was 40 years old, (15 years after the onset of my MS symptoms), I was using a power (electric) wheelchair much of the time. I could still walk with a walker, but it took great effort. Five years later when I moved to Arizona, my walking was limited to about 15 steps and the strain on my upper body was enormous. I decided that it was time to use the power chair full-time, knowing that if I didn't walk anymore, I would lose my ability to do so. The risk of falling down, getting hurt, and breaking something was too great. It would probably throw me into a flare-up; and the rehab for a bad injury or broken bone would not only be an inconvenience, but a physical setback. I wanted to avoid steroids as much as possible because of the increased risk of osteoporosis from using them.

  Using the power chair and scooter full-time actually was wonderful. I had so much less fatigue from not trying to walk and so much more energy to do other things, like swimming more. Swimming was a much more sensible alternative to walking for the following reasons.

- Improves circulation; reduces edema.
- Benefits the respiratory and cardiovascular systems.
- All muscles get a workout for stretching, strengthening and endurance.
- Enables excellent practice for things that are difficult to do on land,
- such as standing, walking, balancing, and improving posture.
- Provides safety from slipping and falling.
- Exercises in cool water are easier.
- Benefits overall health, constipation.
- Relieves stress/provides relaxation.
- Helps burn calories to keep the weight off.

- **I chose not to have another child.**

In the chapter about pregnancy, I described the difficult relapse I had after delivery, and shared my thought process and interchange with my doctor about having a second child. This was devastating for me to accept because I wanted more children very badly, but eventually I worked through it.

I did this by seeking out ways to enjoy other children and being there for those kids who had working mothers. I became the homeroom mother, the soccer mom, the wresting mom, the you-name-it mom by volunteering when I was able to as my son was growing up. Later when I retrained myself in Spanish, I tutored kids for 15 years. I totally loved helping and being there for those kids.

Now, my sister has two girls and I enjoy spoiling them like they were my own grandchildren. It was the right decision for me not to have any more children—I felt the risk was too high for my MS to relapse more frequently.

- **I chose to give up my career.**

  As I mentioned earlier in the chapter about Long-Term Disability, I gave up my career. That was a difficult decision largely because of the impact on our financial situation and the acceptance of the fact that I was giving up all that I had worked for to get to the position I held. The adjustment was huge and took a while. But the amazing thing about that decision was that it actually enabled me to do two things that I had really wanted to do in my life.

  The first was that I was able to be a stay-at-home mom for my son. The second was that I ended up doing what I really wanted to do in my life as a profession, which was to learn Spanish and use it in some way. Though I hate MS, the irony is that I'm not sure I would have enjoyed my life as much if I didn't get it.

- **I chose not to take DMTs.**

  The first three—Avonex, Betaseron, and Copaxone (called the "ABC" drugs) became available in the nineties. At the time, I didn't try them for several reasons—people who came to my MS support group had more negative than positive things to say about them, they were expensive, and I didn't feel comfortable trying new drugs without knowing the long-term effects of them.

  The success rate of these drugs really was unimpressive to me back then. I was following a wellness approach to managing my MS, and was doing very well with that. I preferred to wait it out.

  Since then, I never did try any of these treatments because I don't get many relapses anymore. I'm managing well, despite the damage I've sustained over the years. However, I would never tell someone to not look into them. A person with MS would have to do his/her own research and weigh the benefits vs. the risks/drawbacks as I've mentioned earlier.

- **I chose to get stem cells via IV infusion in the Cayman Islands.**

  As I wrote earlier in the book, I always listen to my body and know it well, but I leave myself open to try something new if I'm confident it is safe. Like everyone else with MS, I want to feel better and get better. There was no desperation when I researched this

140

procedure. My neurologist did not agree with my decision, but my PCP supported me. (I wrote a post about this in the blog section of my website.)

My neurologist suggested I go the HSCT route, but I was adamantly against it. My 32-year-old nephew had leukemia and died in John Hopkins after his bone marrow transplant. (The procedure is relatively the same and has high risk.) He suffered 16 months. So, I flew to Grand Cayman.

All went wonderfully for eight months, and then the improvements began to subside. Today, most of what had improved didn't hold, except for all of the improvements in my troubled hands (as described in the *Invisible Symptoms* chapter).

Did the stem cells play a part? I think so, but will never know for sure. That was two years ago. Yes, I still would do it again. I didn't suffer one minute, and those months were the best I felt in decades. The notes are in my journal.

Note: Earlier, I mentioned that I went to Germany for a treatment that was not available in the U.S. It was 1990, and my MS was extremely aggressive. After thorough research and a supportive nod from my neurologist, I felt safe to go to the clinic and try it. Then, I imported the meds for ten years, and my MS *did* calm down. The other positive to the trip? My husband and I chunked out pieces of the Berlin Wall that was coming down and gave them away as souvenirs!

Words of Inspiration

September 28, 2011

*Life is precious, challenging, and worth getting
out of it what you can.*

Being a lover of American history, one of the items on my bucket list was to visit the actual trail of the Lewis & Clark expedition. As I was returning from an RV road trip with my husband and brother to do this, I wrote this page. During the trip, I reflected on the similarities of their journey and life with MS. This was the final page of the first edition of *Managing MS*.

When Lewis & Clark began their journey to the Pacific Ocean across the continent, they went into unknown territory. Daily they encountered obstacles in the wilderness they had to overcome, and had to rely heavily on the support of each other/ strangers, their skills, ingenuity, and creativity in order to survive and prevail. The team of 33 persons suffered; one died. They experimented. They documented. They learned. They managed and accomplished incredible hardships. There were moments of deep despair and defeat, and moments of high joy and success.

They found their way. I found my way. You will find your way...

The Journey Continues

September 1, 2021

Life is a journey. A distance, course, and area travelled usually over a rather long time.

"Journey" is a word often used to describe someone's life. Sometimes you are joined on that journey. MS joined me early on the road and has been with me ever since.

Knowledge is the engine; support is the battery in my car. Good spark plugs are vital to the engine.

A car that is well taken care of can travel many miles. There is so much to discover and learn when you are on a journey. On the road, lots of help, advice, guidance, and assistance are needed.

Sometimes a car comes to a fork in the road. Sometimes it goes down a dark road. Sometimes it takes a detour. There are many mountains and valleys along the way.

After many miles in the journey, the car starts wearing out, going slower, and needs more maintenance. There are many dents and bruises. Wear and tear from all the miles travelled. But wow, what a ride!

But the car engine is still good, and there is life in the battery. I think this old car will continue the journey. There is so much more to see, learn and experience. A few more bumps, breakdowns and wrong turns won't matter.

Once in a while, the ride gets lonely. Do you want to come along?

I know where I am going. There is no fear of what roadblocks I will encounter, as my journey continues.

After all, I have a mouth and a brain.

Debbie

DEBBIE'S FAVORITE
BLOG POSTS

Brain Health: What to Know, What to do
"Take Care of your Brain"

June 11, 2015

Those affected by Multiple Sclerosis know that MS is a disease of the brain, spinal cord and the optic nerves. When MSers think of their brain, most are concerned about the lesions and possible cognitive impairment. Some people are aware that emotions such as depression and mood swings can also be directly affected by the brain. But I bet most folks don't think or even know that one can take care of their brain to help manage their MS symptoms and progression. **Brain health is a crucial component of one's overall health and wellness.**

As a person who has lived with MS for decades and loves to research, I find myself reading almost daily about the brain. I am equally fascinated both by the tremendous amount of research that has occurred about this complicated organ and what is has been learned about it just in the past few years.

SO HOW DO YOU TAKE CARE OF YOUR BRAIN?

There are many things that can be done specifically for the brain just like one would do for overall wellness: getting enough good sleep, exercise, diet, stress less, etc. that are listed as main categories below. Included are some links to excellent articles from credible sources that expands/explains more information for your knowledge/interests.

- ## Good Sleep: #1 Priority

Sleep affects EVERYTHING in the body—your heart, energy level, pain, weight, and even skin. Your brain cannot function well without it. It affects your mental state: judgment, reaction times, moods, memory, concentration and decision making. Sleep enables your brain to process information and store it in your memory; it rejuvenates parts of your brain that was used during the day and even parts that are not normally used.

Scientists say sleep is nature's panacea, more powerful than any drug in its ability to restore and rejuvenate the human brain and body. Studies consistently show that people who sleep less than eight hours a night don't perform as well on concentration and memory tests. Many people with MS have sleep issues, due to a variety of reasons.

- ## Exercise your Brain

Quite simply, the brain is similar to a muscle—you use it or lose it.

When I was a little girl, my aunt would always tell me to "use my intelligence" for making decisions, solving problems or looking for an answer to something. I was forced to use logic, imagination, creativity and social skills. Television was limited, and my mother made me read every night until I started middle school. They were wise and I was gifted because of it. I yearned to learn and am still doing it.

My cognitive function is now beginning to slip a bit—because of age? MS? menopause? Who knows, but I know there are brain exercises and other things that can be done to help keep my mind sharp.

- ## Diet – "Brain Food"

Yes—there are foods that are specifically good for the brain. And what is good for the brain is also good for the body.

For example, avocados increase blood flow to the brain, and may help in lowering blood pressure. Deep-water fish, such as salmon, are rich in omega-3's and essential fatty acids, which are essential for brain function. Omega-3's also contain anti-inflammatory substances. Turmeric, garlic and cherries have anti-inflammatory properties. Beans stabilize glucose (blood sugar) levels; the brain is dependent on glucose for fuel. Freshly-brewed tea can boost brain power by enhancing memory, focus, and mood. Tea has potent antioxidants that promote healthy blood flow. Check out "Eat Smart for a Healthier Brain", or Google away! http://www.webmd.com/diet/eat-smart-healthier-brain

- **<u>What is good for your heart is good for your brain</u>**

Taking the following steps to keep your heart healthy may also help stave off cognitive decline:

- Don't smoke.
- Sleep 7–8 hours a night.
- Keep your blood pressure and cholesterol levels in check.
- Eat a low-fat, healthy diet.
- Get plenty of exercise.
- Maintain a healthy weight.
- Limit alcohol consumption.
- Get blood sugar levels (and diabetes, if you have it) under control.

While scientists have traditionally viewed brain cells as finite resources, they're now learning that the brain continues regenerating and forming new connections throughout one's life. Although most cognitive reserve is probably built up early in life, engaging in mentally stimulating activities at any age may have a positive effect—and it doesn't have any negative side effects.

- **<u>Stress Less</u>**

It doesn't take a rocket scientist to know that stress affects moods, emotions, concentration and many other parts of the body. Everyone has stress in their lives, but it's the *chronic* stress that will really activate an immune system response—something MSers do not want.

This recent article discusses the implications stress can have on the immune system and change brain chemistry. It is definitely worth a read: "From the Brain to the Immune System, How Stress Pirates Your Whole Body" https://www.yahoo.com/lifestyle/from-the-brain-to-the-immune-system-how-stress-118300620327.html

What de-stresses you? Music? Taking a rest? Talking to a friend? Deep breathing and Yoga? Therapy? Actions to de-stress are critical for your overall wellness, and for managing your MS.

- **Drugs/Medications**

There is no question that all drugs have side effects and work differently for different people—both on the body and the brain. But folks need to do their homework, ask a lot of questions, and weigh the benefits vs. risks of each drug that is taken—both in the short-term and the long-term. In my opinion,

- *You* are in charge ultimately, not your doctor or anyone else.
- *You* know your body best.
- *You* acquire knowledge about the drugs.
- *You* take responsibility for monitoring what you are taking, keeping notes…

It sounds like common sense, but it is amazing how many people don't do these things. One woman I counseled with MS was freaking out about losing her cognitive function. During our conversation, I learned she was taking a sleeping pill, anxiety pills, and pain pills *every* day! Another woman I spoke with last week said her neurologist wanted to start her on a DMT, and she wasn't definitely diagnosed with MS yet!

www.DebbieMS.com (Blog)

Diagnosing Multiple Sclerosis
"What's going on? I'm so scared!"

February 5, 2013

Diagnosing multiple sclerosis is difficult. Being tested and waiting for a diagnosis is grueling for both the patient and their families. Even in this day and age, the process can take months, or even years in some cases. The stress of the testing, office visits and waiting can send someone over the edge.

I often see online posts about this subject, with an added comment like "I'm scared to death..." This always upsets me because someone or some article is not doing the job of explaining an MS diagnosis in an easy-to-understand manner.

Diagnosing Multiple Sclerosis

It takes a long time to get a diagnosis because it is a process of elimination, to rule out other neurological disorders that could be causing the same type of symptoms.

The process begins with a clinical office evaluation, whereby many things can be initially noted, like your history. There are indicators that a good neurologist will check out—such as the Babinski sign (if the bottom of the foot is scraped and the big toe goes up, not down, it is an indication of a neurological disorder.) Other examples? Hyper reflexes, discoloration of the optic nerve in the eye indicating inflammation/optic neuritis, signs of imbalance or incoordination when walking...

150

Next come the numerous tests—MRI's, spinal taps, EVR's, etc. to look for things such as tumors. Many neurological disorders have symptoms that mimic multiple sclerosis like Lyme disease or fibromyalgia. Note: The MRI is a powerful tool, but a neurologist will not only use that particular test for an MS diagnosis as many people like to assume. Why? Because lesions may not show if an MRI is done only on the brain; an MRI should be done on the spinal cord as well to check if lesions are there. Also, sometimes spots on the MRI may look like lesions, but they may be due to another reason.

The term "multiple" in multiple sclerosis is important. Why? *Multiple* symptoms in *multiple* parts of the nervous system have to occur over *multiple* periods of time. My first relapse lasted ten months—I had both sensory and motor disturbances in my left arm and left leg. Mysteriously, all symptoms went away except for a slight residual in my left arm. I didn't have my second relapse until over two years later. That time I went partially blind and I was wetting the bed. When I went back to the neurologist, I was diagnosed immediately! Bingo! —a multiple occurrence in addition to the multiple symptoms in multiple parts of my body.

Finally, a neurologist will most often not give a definite diagnosis until they are definite that it *is* MS.

In the meantime, what should you do while going through this evaluation and waiting game? Try to stay as healthy as possible. Take all measures you can to sleep, eat, reduce stress and keep your resistance up so that you don't get a cold or virus. And know that having multiple sclerosis is not a death sentence or that you will end up in a wheelchair.

A Multiple Sclerosis Diagnosis

Getting an MS diagnosis is extremely frightening. I went through it thirty-two years ago myself, and over the years I have talked to so many people about this as a trained, MS-peer counselor. The fear of the unknown is overwhelming.

Sadly, there are many misconceptions about MS that create a lot of fear. So, for starters, here are some facts to clear up some common ones:

- No, MS is not fatal (though in past decades people died from *complications* of it such as urinary tract problems that led to kidney failure…)

- Although there is no cure, there are treatments available to help symptoms and to slow the relapses/progression of MS.

- It is not congenital (people do not directly inherit MS, though they now know that there is a genetic factor involved.)

- It is not contagious.

- Not everyone ends up in a wheelchair—in the 1980's the estimate was 1 in 4 (25%). Today, statistics are on your side for a better future prognosis, especially with the new treatments available now and the tremendous research that is happening.

So, what should a person do initially when he/she receives a MS diagnosis? These are my recommendations:

- Gain as much knowledge and support from the right places. I suggest starting with the National MS Society and other National MS Associations in the beginning. But there is so much information and so many other resources available it can become overwhelming, confusing and perhaps create more fear. Take baby steps when gathering information.

- Your best source of comfort and information will be from another person who has MS, a peer. However, be selective with whom you talk to and use good judgment. Some unknown people online can cause confusion, be uninformed, misleading, and negative.

- Make sure you have a good neurologist who treats many others with MS or is a MS specialist. You need to trust your doctor and feel comfortable with him/her. Also, make sure that any other specialists that you may need to see (e.g., physical therapist, urologist, etc.) understand MS and have dealt with MS patients.

- Don't panic if you don't get on a treatment right away--it takes time to figure out the right thing to take/do, and waiting won't severely impact your course, for better or for worse. Keep a journal. You will start to see patterns and learn how your body acts and reacts. An easy way to do this is to use a 12-month calendar, with large blocks to jot brief notes in. It is helpful to see patterns when you are looking at a whole month at one time and easier to reference.

- Remember that staying healthy is essential--getting illness/infections could trigger a relapse. MS is an autoimmune disorder; therefore, the immune system is not working properly. When you get sick, you may be twice as sick and it may take twice as long to recover as compared to a "normal" person. Relapses usually result in some residual (damage). It's a must to keep your resistance up—food, sleep, stress management…

Finally, there ARE many things a person can do to manage their MS! **The biggest mistake someone with MS can do is nothing, or expect a shot or a pill to fix everything.** There is no magic pill or shot yet that you can take to make it all go away. It takes work, discipline, dedication, attitude. and the necessity to take care of yourself. MS is still a lifetime illness. Until there is a cure for multiple sclerosis, the goal is to stay healthy, prevent new attacks, and prevent disability.

I am a MS survivor as are so many others! Check out my website for more information.

www.DebbieMS.com (Blog)

Important Things Others Should Know about the Chronically Ill
"An Educating Tool"

July 26, 2014

I was in the middle of writing a blog post about what folks with MS really need from others when I came across this pin I found on Pinterest. What an extraordinary pin to share with my peers!

Because I still look so good after all these years and rarely complain, people around me often forget about my invisible, unpredictable, and interfering symptoms. And it is probably because I am so good at the way I manage this disease. I make it look so easy, when the truth is, it can be a real bitch.

For people who are just learning about how to live with a person with MS or who is chronically ill, a copy of this will be a good, educating tool.

"People with chronic pain and illness want everyone in their lives to know these important things about them…"

1. Don't be upset if I seem on edge. I do the best I can every day to be "normal". I'm exhausted and sometimes I snap.

2. I find it very hard to concentrate at times for a lot of reasons. Pain, drugs, lack of sleep… I'm sorry if I lose focus.

3. Letting my loved ones and friends down by cancelling plans is heartbreaking to me. I want more than anything to be as active as you, and do the things I used to do.

4. My health can change daily. Sometimes hourly. There are a lot of reasons this happens. Weather, stress, flare-ups...I can assure you that I hate it as much as you do.

5. I don't like to whine. I don't like to complain. Sometimes I just need to vent. When this happens, I am not asking for pity or attention. I just need an ear to bend and a hand to hold.

6. During rough times, I find it hard to describe how bad it is. When I say "I'm fine" and you know I am not, it's okay not to ask questions. Just be prepared if the flood gates open because "I'm fine" is often code for "I'm trying to hold it together, but having a rough time. I'm on the edge."

7. If I am hurting bad enough to tell you about it without being asked, please know that it's REALLY bad.

8. When you reach out to me with suggestions to help me feel better, I know that you mean well. If it was as simple as popping a new pill, eating differently or trying a different doctor, I've most likely already tried it and was disappointed.

9. All I truly want from you is friendship, love, support and understanding. It means everything to me.

10. When someone gives me a pep talk, I understand the sentiment. Chronic illness just doesn't go away. I wish it did, too! I appreciate your wanting the best for me, but save the pep talk for the gym or the kids' next volleyball game.

11. It hurts worse than you can possibly imagine when I'm thought of as lazy, unreliable, or selfish. Nothing is further from the truth.

12. I do a lot of silly things to distract myself because any part of my life not consumed with pain is a good part.

13. The simplest tasks can completely drain me. Please know that I do the best I can every day with what I have.

14. Come to me with any questions you may have about my condition. I love you and would much rather tell you about this face to face without judgment.

After all these years I have lived with MS, I may put this on my refrigerator at times. Or, give a copy of this to the forgetful numbskull or insensitive ostrich that has their head in the sand! (Yes, I think we all have a person or two like this in our lives.) And, the next time someone says "What's *wrong* with you?!" I think I will tell them to read #___.

www.DebbieMS.com (Blog)

MS and Your Relationships
"Strategies & Tips"

March 9, 2014

This year I facilitated a workshop entitled "MS and Your Relationships" in Phoenix. The workshop was part of Genzyme's *One Day for Every Day* Event. This is a summary of that workshop, as I want to share this information with a larger audience.

I began by telling the attendees that a two-hour timeframe was not enough for this big, important subject. It's bad enough that everything about MS is complex, from the diagnosis to the symptoms; after all, the nervous system is involved. But people are highly complex too because of their thoughts and emotions. So, when you put the two subjects together—yikes!!

Just about everyone in the room with MS was there with someone else—a spouse, sibling or friend. This was good because *everyone* living with the MSer is also living with MS. And that goes beyond the immediate family.

Genzyme told me to do a presentation on communication strategies and tips to create a foundation of open and honest communication. I adjusted the program to first, make the group interactive, and second, address two other critical aspects of relationships: support and knowledge.

- Support and knowledge reduce the fear one has with an MS diagnosis. The more you have of both, the better chance you have to survive this disease. One has to be careful though where one gets the knowledge since because of social media, there is much information available today that can be overwhelming or misleading.

- Since MS is still a lifetime illness, knowledge and support will change many times as time marches on due to disease progression and lifetime changes that will occur.

- Everyone in the room needs it; everyone outside the room needs it. What is NOT a strategy? Doing nothing—doing no communicating, obtaining no knowledge, getting no support. Anyone dealing with MS will not survive it if none of these are done.

Who are the relationships the person with MS interacts with? What do we say to whom? Who do we need support from?

- Family: partners, children, parents, siblings need communication at appropriate level; "show & tell" is a great game to play to help a non-MSer understand invisible symptoms. For example, have men walk in spike heels to understand balance issues; put 10-lb, weights around ankles to experience walking heaviness and fatigue; put a knit glove on a person and have them find objects in a purse like tissue, quarters, etc.)

- Friends (How much you share depends on depth/closeness of friends.)

- Workplace people: boss, colleagues, human resources (very subjective area—many reasons to disclose or not to disclose)

I asked my audience what groups were missing from the power point slide in the presentation that are just as important?

- Peers (They are a lifeline for both MSers *and* non-MSers—someone you can easily relate to because they are "in your shoes.")

- Healthcare team (Make sure all of them *understand and have experience with persons with MS!* Example, a physical therapist needs to understand the effects of heat and fatigue of MS. You need to *like and trust* your neurologist; if you don't, fire him/her and get another one, as this is a lifetime, crucial relationship.)

- Strangers (I have had to ask strangers for help many times since I had mobility problems since my early years. For example, helping me reach something in a grocery store, or assisting me in a dressing room. People in general--in all of the above groups too--*like and want* to help. It makes them feel good, and they hate to see someone struggle. Personally, I will let people help even if I don't necessarily need it!)

- Pets (Wow—they understand/comfort us the most, don't they?!)

I had all eyes on me from my audience, and many nods or claps. It was interesting to see hands go up when I asked how many felt they needed better support in various groups or who didn't like their neurologist.

Talk is good, even if it doesn't solve anything. It feels good to get things off our chest. I have an old MS buddy who called me recently and asked, "Can you talk to me? Is this a good time?" But if there is someone like a stranger or a fellow employee who asks you something that you don't want to talk about, just simply say: "It's a long story…"

Venting is also good, as long as it doesn't hurt anyone. For example, when I get stressed out or frustrated, I cry or call a close friend of mine who is a peer. My husband on the other hand will yell or throw things in an un-harmful way. We go our separate ways to vent because I don't like his yelling, and he doesn't like my crying. When the steam is released from the pressure cooker, everything calms down. Holding things inside without a release is dangerously stressful, and we all know how stress negatively affects MS.

What if the people we need to talk with will not communicate or talk? Then it is essential to find someone who will…

So, what are strategies to foster healthy communication?

- Should you always be honest about your feelings? When I asked everyone in the room if they were ever *dis*honest about their feelings, every single hand went up! It obviously is a judgment call, depending upon the people involved, and their personalities. With your healthcare team, you need to be honest. With everyone else, the group agreed that you can't be a constant complainer or whiner. Be selective with whom you are comfortable with and trust to discuss your concerns, problems, fears, etc.

- Keep a journal about important things that need to be communicated, whether it is info to discuss with your doctor, modifications that need to be made at work, or just notes about what you want to talk about.

- Pick an appropriate time and place for a discussion. Trying to talk when one is tired, hungry, or stressed out will be a disaster. Try to be in a relaxed frame of mind, when interruptions will not occur.

- Be respectful of what the other person is saying—this is a two-way conversation. Actively listen to each other, and avoid accusations, finger pointing, name calling, yelling, etc. *How* and *what* we say matters, as well as the tone that we use. Avoid negativity.

- Two-thirds of communication occurs through body language. Your posture, facial expressions, eye contact, etc. speaks volumes. When someone rolls their eyes or points a finger at you, what does that indicate?

- Ask *for* help and ask *to* help. People want to help, and people need help. Be explicit or give examples when talking about this to help clarify your statements. Ask questions and share perspectives. Try to put yourself in the other person's shoes. And remember—none of us are mind readers. Not only are you communicating here, you are *educating*.

- Everyone should show and express their gratitude often. Give complements.

- A hug, kiss or smile goes a long way.

- From experience, I believe that we MSers set the tone and comfort level. If we are relaxed and open, the other person will be too.

- My personal advice to all: express *empathy*, not *sympathy*.

160

- Use humor when appropriate. Many times, the subject being discussed can be very sensitive and not funny at all. Or, it is hard to be humorous when you are not feeling well.

- Avoid arguing and be patient. If an argument develops or patience is lost, quit the discussion and regroup later.

- Always try. If it doesn't work, try something else.

We ran way over our two-hour timeframe, which was no surprise. But it was a start, and I always say that "Getting started with anything is the hard part." Now everyone has a framework or some ground rules they can try to use to enhance their communication, support and knowledge.

www.DebbieMS.com (Blog)

The Optimist and the Pessimist
"Attitude is Everything"

August 6, 2014

I am an optimist. My husband is a pessimist. If I say "wow, the sky is so blue", he'll say "I hate the sun, I like it cloudy." They say opposites attract but sometimes I don't know how I have survived 36 years of marriage with a person who is a pessimist.

My husband and I just got back from a mini camping trip in our RV and truthfully, it really was frustrating. It rained constantly for almost the entire trip, so we were confined to stay in the RV. For me, it was cozy listening to the rain while reading a novel and watching movies. For him, he seemed to complain about everything and didn't even want to play cards with me.

After being in this situation, I started writing a post about why the need to vent from time to time is essential to your health. When I took a break, I came across this article about optimism and pessimism in the newspaper. I felt like it was written for me.

This article is so important, I decided to postpone my post and share this instead. Not only is optimism necessary to survive life, it is necessary to survive MS. Pessimistic people drag you down, something that is not good if you are trying to cope with a chronic illness.

Optimism Trumps Pessimism in Workplace, Life

President Harry S. Truman once said, "A pessimist is one who makes difficulties of his opportunities, and an optimist is one who makes opportunities of his difficulties."

Which do you think will reach their goals, live a happy life and achieve their dreams?

Imagine interviewing two people who have identical skills, but one is always grumbling about how unfair life can be, while the other one talks about what wonderful possibilities exist.

Naturally, you would gravitate toward the optimist. If you choose the pessimist, you would be setting yourself up for plenty of aggravation and disappointment, not to mention the negative impact on your staff and customers. Pessimism can bring everyone down, not just the person with the negative attitude.

Pessimism is nothing more than self-sabotage. Expecting only the worst is not being realistic. Realists hope for the best but prepare for the worst. Pessimists can't imagine the best, so they prepare for the worst. And then if the worst never happens? Pessimists often find the worst possible result simply to prove that their concerns were right.

The question becomes, would you rather be right than be happy? That's not being realistic, either. That's being self-defeating. Pessimism can rob you of your energy, sap you of your strength and drain you of your dreams.

Optimism is the remedy. Optimism doesn't mean pretending life is always wonderful. Optimism means embracing reality. You accept that there will be bad days, but also good days. When you're grounded in reality, you know where you are and how far you need to go. Once you know how far your goal may be from where you are, optimism can give you the motivation to make plans to get to where you want to go.

Pessimists see life as one problem after another. Optimists see life as one opportunity after another.

How you look at life can drastically affect how much you enjoy your life. Optimists expect the best out of life.

Does it make sense that pessimists tend to blame others or circumstances for their failures?

Optimists help create some of the good they come to expect, so they are probably right more often than not — and they don't waste time worrying about what they're not right about. Optimism relaxes people. When we're relaxed, there is better blood flow to the brain, which results in more energy and creativity in your life.

There is virtually nothing that you can't do if you set your mind to it. You cannot control events in your life, but you can control how you react.

Do you want to be a pessimist and have no hope for a better future? Or would you rather be an optimist and believe you can achieve a better future?

Mackay's Moral: *Attitude is the mind's paintbrush — it can color any situation.*

Harvey Mackay is the author of the New York Times best-seller "Swim With the Sharks Without Being Eaten Alive." He can be reached through his website, harveymackay.com

In my situation, I learned years ago how to ignore or escape my husband's negativity. While I succeeded most of the time, the times that I couldn't get away from it caused tremendous stress. Not only did the stress intensify my MS symptoms, it would cause me to be moody and stifle my motivation to move forward.

Fortunately, I am a strong-willed person and almost always found alternative sources of optimism (e.g., friends, enjoyable interests/activities…) to lift me up before I got dragged into the depths of an abyss.

Now, in all fairness, my husband is a great guy and has many positive attributes. None of us is perfect. I am a sensitive person who cries easily or pouts. Personality traits are difficult to change; a person has to recognize a change needs to be made and then take great effort to make the changes. But this is a slow process that requires much patience.

An optimist living with a pessimist will be a lethal combination if coping mechanisms can't be accomplished.

I know from experience. And I know that one of the main reasons I have survived managing my MS is because I am an optimist. Attitude is everything.

www.DebbieMS.com (Blog)

The Truth about MS and Wheelchairs
"My Personal Insights"

———————————

September 5, 2014

If you asked anyone "What do you think of when you hear the term MS?" the answer usually includes "wheelchairs".

When my first relapse happened back in 1980, a picture of a person with MS in a wheelchair was always shown, even by the MS Society. Perhaps it was to help with fundraising, or perhaps it **was to a way** to draw attention to a disease that was not usually heard of.

Whatever the case, it did create a picture of "*This* is MS" and the huge fear of living a life in a wheelchair. That vision still exists today, despite the advances in awareness and research that have occurred. Despite the reality that MS involves many other neurological symptoms in addition to a life in a wheelchair.

I know much about this because I am one of those MSers who ended up in a wheelchair. And I want to speak up about MS and wheelchairs to try to correct that picture and reduce that fear for anyone dealing with MS.

1. **Over a lifetime, only 20-25% end up in a wheelchair.** That was the statistic in 1980, and it probably is less today due to the development of the disease-modifying drugs that have been available since the mid-90's. *

   I have many friends who have had MS over 30 years, and I am the one of a few who is in a wheelchair permanently. Now, of course many patients use walkers or canes since MS and mobility problems usually go hand-in-hand; but most are not hunched over, paralyzed, and completely debilitated in a wheelchair.

*Note: This statistic is listed in many reputable resources. The National MS Society used to use this percentage, but changed it to 35% based on some study. I question their revision and the study. With the numerous DMTs that have been/are available, the percentage of MSers in wheelchairs permanently should have declined, not increased.

2. **A person can have a quality life living in a wheelchair, though admittedly the limitations it causes can be frustrating.** Again, I know.

   I manage my MS well and despite having lived permanently in a wheelchair these past thirteen years, I have had a happy life. I travel, swim, volunteer, take care of many household responsibilities... And the other MSers I know who are in my position would agree their lives are full and active.

   Having MS certainly is not a cakewalk, but it certainly isn't the end of the world either. There are far worse things in life. Plus, I must add that there are other MS symptoms that can be extremely difficult, such as vision loss and overwhelming fatigue. However, so many of these symptoms can be successfully managed to minimize their interfering effects.

3. **Wheelchairs should be viewed as a friend, not the enemy.** So, you ask, what the heck does THAT mean? I'll explain.

   At many MS events and online, I see and hear people with mobility issues struggling with trying to walk without a walking aid, or one that is not suitable for them. Part of it is due to vanity, or part of it is a desire to not "give in" to MS.

   - Is vanity worth the risk of falling down and getting hurt? In truth, I purposely started using a wheelchair full-time even though I could walk with a walker for 15-30 steps. The years on steroids, the osteoporosis, and my age put me at great risk for breaking an arm or leg. Instead, I used the swimming pool to walk and exercise safely.

- Before I went into the chair permanently, I used a power chair on a part-time basis around the house and scooters that were available in stores for customers. It is a tremendous help in reducing fatigue and getting more things done. This was a great morale booster. In addition, the pain from overused muscles and poor posture was lessoned substantially.

- I wasn't giving into my MS at all. Wheelchairs *enabled* me. There are many persons with MS that will use a scooter or wheelchair because of fatigue, weakness, balance problems, or to assist with conserving energy.

Before I decided to post this article, I talked to a couple of good friends of mine to ask them about the content of this article. They, like me, are "Ol' MS Vets", i.e., those who have lived with MS for decades and also have been involved with the MS community.

www.DebbieMS.com (Blog)

RESOURCES/ BIBLIOGRAPHY

MS Blogs/Newsletters/Forums

MS Views and News / Stu's Views & MS News
Provides education, information & resources for those affected
by Multiple Sclerosis
www.msviewsandnews.org

ActiveMSers
Is designed to help, motivate, & inspire those with multiple sclerosis to
stay as active as possible - physically, intellectually and socially -
regardless of physical limitations.
www.activemsers.org

MS Fitness Challenge
Encouraging People to Overcome Multiple Sclerosis Through Fitness
and Nutrition
http://msfitnesschallenge.com/

MS Conversations
Register to stay informed on all the latest MS News, participate in
forums...
https://blog.mymsaa.org/author/multiplesclerosis.net/

MultipleSclerosis.net
https://multiplesclerosis.net/

MS News Today
https://multiplesclerosisnewstoday.com/

MS Healthline
https://ms.healthline.com/

Momentum Magazine
https://bit.ly/3hDBB24

The Motivator Magazine
https://mymsaa.org/publications/motivator/

International Journal of MS Care
https://meridian.allenpress.com/ijmsc

Yvonne deSousa
http://yvonnedesousa.com/blog/
Author of *MS Madness*

Nicole Lemelle
http://www.mynewnormals.com/

Articles

My MS Manager™, the first-of-its kind mobile phone app
created by the Multiple Sclerosis Association of America (MSAA) to
help patients with MS better manage their disease

Exercising with MS: The Complete Guide
ActiveMSers – Dave Bexfield

Tips to Manage Your Muscles
http://www.webmd.com/multiple-sclerosis/live-thrive-16/feel-
best/muscles

Spasticity--What it is & what to do
https://multiplesclerosis.net/symptoms/stiffness-involuntary-muscle-
spasms/

Stretching for People with MS
https://www.nationalmssociety.org/NationalMSSociety/media/MSNationalFiles/Brochures/Brochure-Stretching-for-People-with-MS.pdf

Expanded Disability Status Scale (EDSS)
http://bit.ly/1pmf0Ge

Multiple Sclerosis by the Numbers: Facts, Statistics, and You"
http://bit.ly/SbztzP

Bowel Changes in MS
https://www.ms.org.au/attachments/bowel-handouts-merged-2015.aspx

What is a Neurogenic Bowel?
https://www.saintlukeskc.org/health-library/neurogenic-bowel

How to Treat a Fecal Impaction
https://www.medicalnewstoday.com/articles/322150

How temperature affects people with Multiple Sclerosis
http://brainblogger.com/2014/09/13/how-temperature-affects-people-with-multiple-sclerosis/

How to Boost Your Immune System
http://bit.ly/19huu2H

The Power of Sleep
http://time.com/3326565/the-power-of-sleep/

The Complete Guide to Insomnia and How You Can Manage It
https://howtosleep.co.uk/guides/the-complete-guide-to-insomnia

Solutions for Cooling Every Body
http://www.polarproducts.com/polarshop/pc/home.asp

Americans with Disabilities Act/Legal/Employment

- ADA Guide:
  https://www.ada.gov/cguide.htm#anchor62335

- ADA & People with MS | Employment Issues
  http://bit.ly/1uBj60V

- Know Your Rights: A Legal Guide for People Living with Multiple
  Sclerosis
  http://www.nationalmssociety.org/Programs-and-
  Services/Resources/Know-Your-Rights-A-Legal-Guide-for-
  People-Living-w?page=1&orderby=3&order=asc

- Disclosing MS On the Job: Why I Did, and Why I Didn't
  (11/17/2020)
  https://multiplesclerosis.net/living-with-ms/disclosing-job-work-
  reasons/

  Useful site:
  Job Accommodation Network (JAN)
  https://askjan.org/

Associations: Multiple Sclerosis

- National Multiple Sclerosis Society (NMSS)
  www.nationalmssociety.org
  1-800-344-4867

- Multiple Sclerosis Association of America (MSAA)
  www.mymsaa.org
  1-(800) 532-7667

- Multiple Sclerosis Foundation (MSF)
  www.msfocus.org
  1- 888-MSFOCUS

- Multiple Sclerosis International Federation
  http://www.msif.org/en/

- The Consortium of Multiple Sclerosis Centers
  The leading educational and professional development organization for MS healthcare professionals.
  http://www.mscare.org/

- iConquorMS - a Patient-Powered Research Network (PPRN)
  https://www.iconquerms.org/

- MSology is a free information service offering the latest research news on multiple sclerosis (MS), tips on living with the disease, and practical advice to help in making decisions.
  http://msology.ca/

- WEGO Health (for Patient Leaders)
  https://www.wegohealth.com/

- Shift MS
  https://shift.ms/

Associations: Other

- Myelin Repair Foundation
  info@myelinrepair.org
  http://www.myelinrepair.org
  Tel: 408-871-2410

- Well Spouse Association
  http://www.wellspouse.org
  Tel: 800-838-0879 732-577-8899

- Caregiving Resource Center--Information, tools and tips for caregivers (AARP)
  http://bit.ly/1yFBnMV

Doctors: Background Check (Profiles, Credentials, Ratings, Reviews)

- www.healthgrades.com
- www.vitals.com

Handicapped Placard/License Plates

To get a handicapped or license plate, contact the motor vehicle department in your state for qualifications and forms.

Healthcare/Insurance Information

- Agency for Healthcare Research & Quality: Patient & Consumer Services
  http://www.ahrq.gov/patients-consumers/index.html

- Healthcare Coverage: FAQ'S
  https://www.healthcare.gov/all-topics/

- U.S. Department of Health and Human Services
  Affordable Care Act; Prevention/wellness; other HHS info
  http://www.hhs.gov/healthcare/index.html

- Evaluating Health Information—MedlinePlus
  Lots of health information swirling around out there. How can you tell what's legit? Check out this resource for guidance.
  http://www.nlm.nih.gov/medlineplus/evaluatinghealthinformation.html

General Healthcare/Mental Health/Alternative Medicine/Pain Management

- Benefits of Tai Chi for MS
  https://www.healthcentral.com/article/benefits-of-tai-chi-for-multiple-sclerosis … MultipleSclerosis

- Coping with Stress Manual, along with a Guided Imagery Audio Track. This manual will help individuals and their families to cope with stress.
  https://app.box.com/s/k49hidmxdohdmvg3p2bx83v4rxydntnj

- Preventing Abuse and Multiple Sclerosis
  https://www.mymsteam.com/resources/preventing-abuse-and-multiple-sclerosis

- Forms of Emotional and Verbal Abuse You May Be Overlooking
  https://www.psychologytoday.com/us/blog/toxic-relationships/201704/forms-emotional-and-verbal-abuse-you-may-be-overlooking

- Dealing with Emotional Abuse
  https://bit.ly/2TP2iaE

- National Domestic Violence hotline 1-800-799-7233
  https://www.domesticshelters.org/

- Emotionally Abusive Men and Women: Who Are They?
  https://www.healthyplace.com/abuse/emotional-psychological-abuse/emotionally-abusive-men-and-women-who-are-they

- Free Online Therapy Services-- mental health support offered is secure, reliable, and developed for all types of patients
  https://www.onlinetherapy.com/free

- Health Risk & Fitness Assessments/Calculators
  http://www.calculators.org/health/

- Healthline—a health and wellness information site
  http://www.healthline.com/

- Positive Health and Wellness—this site has a variety of info to live a more positive, healthier, happy life
  https://www.positivehealthwellness.com

- Drug-Free Remedies for Chronic Pain
  http://www.aarp.org/health/alternative-medicine/info-11-2008/drug_free_remedies_chronic_pain.html

Medical Information

- American Academy of Neurology
  American Brain Foundation
  https://www.americanbrainfoundation.org/

- Drugs.com
  This site provides accurate and independent information on more than 24,000 prescription drugs, over-the-counter medicines & natural products.
  https://www.drugs.com/

- Drug-Nutrient Interactions and Drug-Supplement Interactions | What You Need to Know
  http://bit.ly/1xdavm7
  www.drugwatch.com/health/
  www.drugwatch.com/drugs-and-devices/

- FDA List of Vaccines
  http://www.fda.gov/BiologicsBloodVaccines/Vaccines/Approved Products/ucm093833.htm

- Medical Dictionary
  Descriptions of medical conditions, medications, anatomical terms, etc. are provided in this website.
  www.thefreedictionary.com (click "Medical Dictionary")

- MedlinePlus is the National Institutes of Health's Web site for patients and their families and friends. Produced by the National Library of Medicine, information is given about diseases, conditions, etc. in language easily understood. MedlinePlus offers reliable, up-to-date health information, free.
  www.nlm.nih.gov/medlineplus

- WebMD
  Provides health information, tools for managing your health, and support to those who seek information. The content is timely and credible.
  www.webmd.com

- MS Research Update
  The 2020 edition is a comprehensive overview of research findings on the FDA-approved disease-modifying therapies, as well as many experimental treatments
  https://mymsaa.org/publications/msresearch-update-2020

Other Resources

- Advance Medical Directives (Living Wills, Power of Attorney, Health Care Proxy)
  https://www.medicinenet.com/advance_medical_directives/articl e.htm

- Compassion and Choices - Life/Care Planning and End-of-Life Options
  1-800-247-7421 https://compassionandchoices.org/

- Care Options and Programs-- comprehensive information to maintain independence & quality of life, (State or National)
  https://www.caring.com/senior-living/assisted-living/arizona

- Guide on Financial Assistance and Funding for Assisted Living and Senior Care
  https://www.payingforseniorcare.com/longtermcare/paying-for-assisted-living.html

Social Security Disability Benefits/Medicare

To obtain information about Social Security Disability, you can call your local social security office, or go online at www.socialsecurity.gov.

Another very informative site for this subject is www.NMSS.org (Type "social security disability" in the search bar.)

- Social Security Disability Benefits Guide
  http://www.thesimpledollar.com/disability-benefits-guide/

- A Guide to Medicare Benefits
  https://www.caring.com/medicare/

- Social Security Disability Benefit Calculator
  http://www.thesimpledollar.com/disability-benefits-guide/#social-security-disability-benefit-calculator

- Social Security Disability Law Updates for the MS Community (Excellent Video)
  https://bit.ly/2UREzqU

Suicide Hotline

The U.S. National Suicide Prevention Lifeline at 800-273-TALK (8255), is a free, 24/7 service that can provide suicidal persons or those around them with support, information and resources. (Source: National Institute of Mental Health.)

Support

- MS Friends
  http://www.nationalmssociety.org/Resources-Support/Find-Support/Connect-with-Peers-One-on-One

- Call 2-1-1
  Similar to dialing 9-1-1 for emergencies, calling 2-1-1 helps people seeking training, employment, food pantries,

- Multiple Sclerosis Discovery Forum
  An online community and information portal that aims to inspire connections and clinical advances
  http://www.msdiscovery.org/

Treatments (DMT)

- <u>Disease Modifying Therapies (DMT's) and Other Medications</u>
  https://www.nationalmssociety.org/Treating-MS/Medications#section-1

- <u>Stem Cells in MS</u>
  https://www.nationalmssociety.org/Research/Research-News-Progress/Stem-Cells-in-MS

- <u>DVC Stem</u> offers cell infusion and other treatments for MS at their Medical Center in the Cayman Islands. Protocols are IRB approved, and the cells come from regulated, U.S. based, FDA compliant laboratories. Treatment consists of a two-day period including the IV transplant of 300M cord tissue-derived MSCs, as well as a variety of therapies designed to aid stem cell activation and potency (chiro, physiotherapy, acupuncture, lymphatic massage, etc.)
  https://www.dvcstem.com/

ABOUT THE AUTHOR

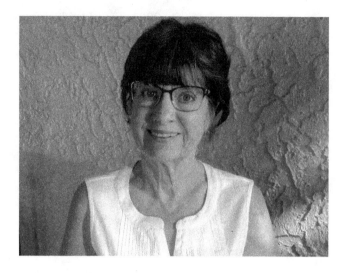

During the past four decades that Debbie Petrina lived with MS, she has spoken to thousands of persons affected by MS—in social media, as a trained peer counselor, and as a participant in numerous events for the NMSS, MS community and other institutions. She earned her B.S. in B.A. degree ('76) from Duquesne University, Pittsburgh, PA. Skills used from her early banking career in finance/research, sales and management have been invaluable as she engaged herself with MS and its community.

Debbie published Managing MS in 2011 and established her website www.DebbieMS.com to help others understand and deal with multiple sclerosis. Much has happened and changed as her MS journey continued, inspiring Debbie to write an enhanced, second edition. She has always strived to reduce fears associated with MS through practical knowledge and support. An avid reader, volunteer, and swimmer, Debbie currently resides in Glendale, AZ with her husband, Dennis and dogs, Grizzly and

Denali. Her ability to effectively manage her MS enables her to maintain independence and enjoy travelling in their accessible RV.

A note from Debbie

Thank you for purchasing and reading my book. I am extremely grateful and hope you found value in reading it. Please consider sharing it with friends or family and leaving a review online. Your feedback and support are always appreciated, and allow me to continue doing what I love.

CPSIA information can be obtained
at www.ICGtesting.com
Printed in the USA
LVHW100110290622
722328LV00004B/307